Questions and Answers for the UKCAT

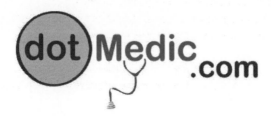

Questions and Answers for the UKCAT

Stephen Seale
BM BCh (Oxon) MA (Cantab), nMRCGP
GP Principal in Cornwall

and

Sam Radford
BM BCh (Oxon) MA (Oxon), nMRCGP
GP Principal in Cornwall

and

Noor Hamad
BM BCH (Oxon) MA (Cantab), nMRCGP, MRCP
GP in Cornwall

© dotMedic Ltd, 2014

ISBN 978 1 907904 51 6

First published 2014

---

dotMedic Limited
Floral Cottage, Mithian, St Agnes, Cornwall, TR5 0QQ

www.dotMedic.com

Important Note from the Publisher
The information in this book was obtained by dotMedic Ltd from what are believed to be reliable sources. Every effort has been made ensure the accuracy of this information, however no responsibility for loss or injury whatsoever occasioned to any person acting or refraining from action as a result of information contained herein can be accepted by the authors or publishers.

Although every effort has been made to ensure that all owners of copyright material have been acknowledged in this book, we would be pleased to acknowledge any omissions brought to our attention in subsequent reprints or editions.

Registered names, trademarks, etc. used in this book, even when not marked as such, are not considered to be protected by law.

Printed in the UK

CONTENTS:

Preface

UKCAT stands for United Kingdom Clinical Aptitude Test and is sat by the majority of candidates who are applying to study medicine, dentistry or veterinary medicine in the UK. There are so many good candidates with excellent grades and work experience that this exam has been formed to help universities decide who to accept. Whether it works effectively or not is the subject of debate, but the reality remains that this exam has become one more hoop that future professionals have to jump through. It is not a great hurdle, but is one that requires familiarity and plenty of practice in order to excel.

Factual knowledge is not assessed in the UKCAT. The main thrust of the exam is aimed at making candidates think quickly under pressure. Given unlimited time, most candidates would be able to score highly. The trick therefore lies in familiarizing oneself with the questions types and practising questions under timed conditions. This book aims to do this by providing explanations of the different question types, example questions to work through step-by-step and further questions to practise under timed conditions. Full explanations are provided for every question and there are hints and tips sections to help you improve your score. Information regarding how, where and when the exam is taken and how different universities use your score is also provided.

A small number of universities, including Oxford, Cambridge, Imperial College and University College London, use a different test known as the BioMedical Admissions Test (BMAT). BMAT is not covered in this book. However, if you are applying to multiple universities, the likelihood is that you will have to sit the UKCAT for at least a couple of your chosen universities. If you are not sure you should check individual university websites for the latest requirements for application.

Medicine, dentistry and veterinary medicine are all highly rewarding careers. We hope you find this book useful and wish you the best of luck in your application.

Further practice questions and exams are available at www.dotmedic.com using the unique code found within this book.

Dr Stephen Seale BM BCh MRCGP
Dr Noor Hamad BM BCh MRCGP MRCP
Dr Samuel Radford BM BCh MRCGP

General Information

The UKCAT is designed to try and provide a means of identifying candidates with the most suitable skills to become future professionals. It has been divided in to five sections; four of these are used to determine your score. These are verbal reasoning, quantitative reasoning, abstract reasoning and decision analysis. Situational judgment is the final part of the exam and considered a measure of 'non-cognitive attributes' and you will be 'banded' depending on how well your answers match to those of a panel of experts.

Verbal reasoning:

This is designed to 'assess the ability to critically evaluate information that is presented in a written form'. You are required to read a short passage of about 200 words and then answer four questions relating to it. There are 11 passages and a total of 44 questions to be completed in 21 minutes (and one minute to read the instructions).

Quantitative reasoning:

This is designed to 'assess the ability to critically evaluate information presented in a numerical form.' You are given numerical information in the form of prose, tables or graphs and then asked four questions relating to the data. There are a total of 36 questions to be completed in 24 minutes (and one minute to read the instructions)

Abstract reasoning:

This is designed to 'assess the ability to change track, critically evaluate and generate hypotheses and requires you to query judgements as you go along.' You are required to identify patterns in sets of shapes. There are a total of 55 questions to be completed in 13 minutes (and one minute to read the instructions).

Decision analysis:

This is designed to 'assess the ability to make sound decisions and judgements using complex information.' You are asked to solve codes and give the most appropriate translation. There are 28 questions relating to the code to be completed in 31 minutes (and one minute to read the instructions).

There is currently (2013/14) a trial of the use of confidence ratings in this part of the test. The results of this will not count as part of your score and will not be communicated to universities. You will be asked to rate on a scale from 1 (not confident) to 5 (very confident) how sure you are you have the correct answer.

Situational Judgment Test:

This assesses 'judgment regarding situations encountered in the workplace.' You are asked to decide how you would respond in certain scenarios. There are 67 questions to be done in 26 minutes (and one minute to read the instructions). This part of the test does NOT count towards your final numerical score but you are assigned a 'band' showing how well you answered the questions. Universities then vary in how and whether they use this score.

Overview of the UKCAT

Section	Items	Standard Test Time	Extended Test Time
Verbal Reasoning	44	22 minutes	28 minutes
Quantitative Reasoning	36	25 minutes	31.5 minutes
Abstract Reasoning	55	14 minutes	17.5 minutes
Decision Analysis	28	32 minutes	39 minutes
Situational Judgement	67	27 minutes	34 minutes
Total		120 minutes	150 minutes

Sitting the UKCAT

When?

You need to sit the UKCAT between the beginning of July and early October and are able to register from early May.

Top tips: Book early and don't leave the exam until the last minute. Exam centres often fill up quickly and you may end up travelling a long way!
Also, don't take the test if you get ill. You will be allowed to reschedule as long as you give enough notice. If you miss the exam don't panic - you are allowed to rebook but will have to pay again.

Where?

You can take the exam at Pearson Vue centres that are found throughout the UK. It is also possible to sit the test outside the UK.

How?

Registration is done via the UKCAT website, www.ukcat.ac.uk. First, create an online account. You will then be emailed a password that allows you to book the test. Currently, the test costs £65 if taken between 1st July and 31st August. From 1st September to 4th October the cost is £80. Sitting it outside the EU is more expensive, at £100.

Top tip: Ask for extra time if you are allowed it – this can be arranged for candidates with special educational needs such as dyslexia or attention deficit disorder.

On The Day

Wake up at least 2-3 hours before you are due to sit the test. Make sure you know how you are going to get to the test centre, exactly where it is and, if necessary, where you can park.

Don't forget your ID! In the UK, you are required to bring current valid photographic identification, such as an original signed passport or photo-card driving license.

Arrive early (at least 15 minutes before your test is scheduled) and register and show your ID.

Top tip: Remember you are not allowed to take anything in to the test room with you. An onscreen calculator is available and you will be given a booklet containing three laminated note boards and a permanent marker pen to make notes with.

In The Exam

Don't spend too long on individual questions. Be strict about moving on and if you have time at the end come back to ones you have flagged. It's probably best to guess an answer before you move on, as you may not have time to come back to look at 'flagged' questions.

Use the ear protectors to cut out all background noise and get yourself 'in the zone'.

Stay calm and focused and remember you have an advantage because you have read this book!

Top tip: Always give an answer to every question, even if you have not had time to read the question. There is no negative marking and by guessing you are likely to be lucky 20-25% of the time.

Results

As you leave the test centre you will be given a copy of your result and should keep this for your records. There is no 'pass mark' for the UKCAT. Individual sections of the UKCAT are marked out of 900 and different universities use the result in different ways. Your mark should help you decide which universities to apply for, as universities publish on their websites how they use the test. Make sure you consider that information and the score you have when you decide which to apply to.

Examples of how your result may be used include:

Overall average in the whole exam above a certain mark (for example 70%).

All sections of the exam require scores above a certain mark.

A requirement for candidates to be in the top 50% of candidates sitting the UKCAT to be considered for an offer.

Further Information

www.ukcat.ac.uk is the official website and the most up to date information and further practice questions can be found there. We recommend you do all of these and also the further practice questions available at www.dotmedic.com

Further details regarding how each university uses the UKCAT score is available on individual university websites.

Chapter 1

Verbal Reasoning

Verbal reasoning

What is it?

UKCAT says: 'The verbal reasoning subtest assesses your ability to read and think carefully about information presented in passages and to determine whether specific conclusions can be drawn from the information presented. You are not expected to use prior knowledge to answer the questions.'

In the verbal reasoning part of the test you are provided with 11 reading passages of approximately 300 words each. There are 4 questions relating to each passage and you must read the instructions and answer a total of 44 questions in 22 minutes.

There are two types of questions:

Type 1: You must decide whether four statements relating to the passage are 'true', 'false' or that you 'can't say'. These are likely to form the majority of the questions.

Type 2: From a choice of four statements about the passage, you must decide which is 'true'. Other questions may be 'which is most likely to be true?', 'most likely to be false?' or 'is false?'. There will probably be fewer of this type of question in the test.

The passages can be on any subject so you cannot (and should not!) revise for them. Only use the information within the text to formulate your answer. Remember the test is looking at how well you can interpret written information, not at what you already know.

Why is verbal reasoning included in the test?

Throughout any professional career you will be required to 'critically appraise' information you are given. This means that you should be able to understand, interpret and draw correct deductions from information in whatever form it comes. This may be via media such as television, books, journals or the internet, or from spoken information from patients or other professionals. Good critical appraisal of information includes the ability to keep an open mind, differentiate between opinion and fact, make value judgments and always considering alternative explanations. Very little is as it first appears - there is always more to the story!

Top Tips:

- *Read the passage quickly once to gain an overall view of the subject. This should take about 40 seconds and there may be bits you need to go back to later to clarify. All you are trying to do here is to get a good idea of what the passage is about and where relevant information lies within it.*
- *Use only information given to you in the passage and don't use any of your own knowledge to help you answer questions (see examples)*
- *The answer to a particular statement is often held in just one of the paragraphs. If this is the case, re-read that paragraph again carefully to check your answer. Skim the rest of the text to check there is nothing else that contradicts it.*
- *If you cannot find a quick answer and are running out of time, the chances are that the answer '**Can't tell**' may be correct. Generally it is easier to write ambiguous statements and if the answer is not quickly obvious 'Can't tell' is a good bet.*

Type 2 questions:

- If you are asked to choose between statements, it is usually easy to rule out one or two of the answers. Then focus your effort on the remaining statements.
- It takes longer to answer these questions and it is easier to get 'bogged down'. Be strict with your time-keeping. If you struggle with these, it may be worth leaving them until last.
- If you get stuck, try and decide whether each statement is true, false or 'can't tell' as you would for the usual questions

Remember to:

- **Answer ALL the questions - THERE IS NO NEGATIVE MARKING**.

- Ask yourself whether statements are presented as opinions or facts. If they are opinions, then it is very likely there are other possibilities and the answer is likely to be 'Can't tell'

- Only answer true or false if it is explicitly said or can be implied from the text that this is the case. Answer 'can't tell' if you are in doubt.

- Understand the meanings of words that have specific implications of frequency or possibility.

- **Never**, **impossible** and **cannot** all imply that something does not happen. These are used in definite statements and can signify that any statement

3

containing these words will be true or false.

- **Similarly**, **always** and **invariably** imply that something happens without leaving any possibility of anything else. Again, use of these words tends to signify statements will be either true or false.

- **Can**, **could**, **may** and **might** imply possibility but not frequency. For example, 'People **can** ski to the South Pole' means it is possible, but you cannot tell how often it happens. Similarly 'I **might** fall off my bike today' does not mean that it is likely (or unlikely) to happen.

- **Usually**, **mostly** and **generally** all imply that something occurs 'most of the time' and this can be taken to be more than 50% cases.

- **Often**, **frequently** and **commonly** imply that something is not unusual. However, this is not necessarily more than 50% of the time.

- **Occasionally** implies that something does not occur often (less than 50% of the time) but more often than **infrequently**, **rarely**, **seldom** or **uncommonly** which all imply that something is unusual but still may occur.

If you decide a statement is true, this means that the statement is either directly made in the passage or logically implied. *Even if you know the statement to be true from your general knowledge, if it is not in or implied by the passage then you cannot say it is true.*

If you decide a statement is false, this means information in the passage contradicts the statement or logically implies it is not true. Again, *if you know the statement to be false from your general knowledge, only mark it as false if you are able to tell this from the information given in the passage.*

If you decide you cannot tell whether the statement is true of false, this means there is insufficient information in the passage for you to be able to give a definitive answer. The statement 'could possibly be true' or 'could possibly be false' – you simply 'can't tell' for certain!

Worked Examples:

Example 1

The Internet and the World Wide Web

Many people use the terms Internet and World Wide Web, or just the Web, interchangeably, but the two terms are not synonymous. The World Wide Web is a global set of documents, images and other resources, logically interrelated by hyperlinks and referenced with Uniform Resource Identifiers (URIs). URIs symbolically identify services, servers and other databases, and the documents and resources that they can provide. Hypertext Transfer Protocol (HTTP) is the main access protocol of the World Wide Web, but it is only one of the hundreds of communication protocols used on the Internet. Web services also use HTTP to allow software systems to communicate in order to share and exchange business logic and data.

World Wide Web browser software, such as Microsoft's Internet Explorer, Mozilla Firefox, Opera, Apple's Safari and Google Chrome, lets users navigate from one web page to another via hyperlinks embedded in the documents. These documents may also contain any combination of computer data, including graphics, sounds, text, video, multimedia and interactive content that runs while the user is interacting with the page. Client-side software can include animations, games, office applications and scientific demonstrations. Through keyword-driven Internet research using search engines like Yahoo! and Google, users worldwide have easy, instant access to a vast and diverse amount of online information. Compared to printed media, books, encyclopaedias and traditional libraries, the World Wide Web has enabled the decentralisation of information on a large scale.

The Web has also enabled individuals and organisations to publish ideas and information to a potentially large audience online at greatly reduced expense and time delay. Publishing a web page, a blog, or building a website involves little initial cost and many cost-free services are available. Publishing and maintaining large, professional web sites with attractive, diverse and up-to-date information is still a difficult and expensive proposition, however.

(Adapted from wikipedia, the free online encyclopaedia. http://en.wikipedia.org/wiki/Internet)

Decide whether the following statements are 'true', 'false' or that you 'can't tell':

Statement 1:

'All world wide web browser software enables users to navigate using hyperlinks' CT

Scanning the document quickly, it becomes clear there is a lot of technical information which is not easy to understand.

The information is presented as fact rather than opinion, so we should take it as such.

This statement clearly relates to the beginning of the second paragraph.

Re-reading this, several examples of browser software that enable users to navigate using hyperlinks are given. For these, we know the statement is true.

However, the statement relates to 'all' browsers and it is possible that some don't enable navigation using hyperlinks. Even if we know this not to be the case from our own knowledge, we cannot imply that the statement is definitely true for all browsers and must therefore answer **'can't tell'**.

Statement 2:

'Information has become more readily available following the invention of the internet'

Common knowledge tells us this is true. However, it is important to check that this is stated or implied in the passage. This is the case in the second paragraph: 'Through keyword-drive internet research… users worldwide have easy, instant access to a vast amount of online information. The answer is therefore **'true'**.

Statement 3:

'Most people in the World have access to the internet'

Another quick scan of the paragraph confirms that there is no explicit phrase that suggests this to be either true or false. The answer is therefore **'can't tell'**.

Statement 4:

'HTTP is often used for access the World Wide Web'

HTTP is only mentioned in the first paragraph, when it is stated that 'HTTP is the main access protocol of the World Wide Web'. The statement is therefore '**true**'.

If the statement had used 'usually' or 'most often' then the answer would not have been so clear and we would have had to answer 'can't tell'. This is because 'usually' and 'most often' imply more than 50% and although we know that HTTP is the 'main' access protocol, it's debatable as to whether 'main' is more than 50%. In these less clear cases, 'can't tell' is the safer answer.

Example 2:

Outer Space

Outer space, or simply space, is the void that exists between celestial bodies including the Earth. It is not completely empty, but consists of a hard vacuum containing a low density of particles: predominantly a plasma of hydrogen and helium, as well as electromagnetic radiation, magnetic fields and neutrinos. Observations have recently proven that it also contains dark matter and dark energy. The baseline temperature, as set by the background radiation left over from the Big Bang is only 2.7 kelvin (K); in contrast, temperatures in the coronae of stars can reach over a million kelvin. Plasma with an extremely low density (less than one hydrogen atom per cubic meter) and high temperature (millions of kelvin) in the space between galaxies accounts for most of the baryonic (ordinary) matter in outer space; local concentrations have condensed into stars and galaxies. Intergalactic space takes up most of the volume of the Universe, but even galaxies and star systems consist almost entirely of empty space.

There is no firm boundary where space begins. However the Karman line, at an altitude of 100 km (62 mi) above sea level, is conventionally used as the start of outer space for the purpose of space treaties and aerospace records keeping. The framework for international space law was established by the Outer Space Treaty, which was passed by the United Nations in 1967. This treaty precludes any claims of national sovereignty and permits all states to explore outer space freely. In 1979, the Moon treaty made the surfaces of objects such as planets, as well as the orbital space around these bodies, the jurisdiction of the international community. Additional resolutions regarding the peaceful uses of outer space have been drafted by the United Nations, but these have not precluded the deployment of weapons into outer space, including the live testing of anti-satellite weapons.

(Adapted from Wikipedia, the free online encyclopaedia http://en.wikipedia.org/wiki/Outer_space)

Question 1

Which of the following statements is least likely to be true?

- Background radiation can influence temperature
- All nations are committed to the United Nation's goal of a peaceful Outer Space
- The Outer Space Treaty has been a success
- Stars and galaxies are thought to have formed from plasma

Answer: 'All nations have committed to the United Nation's goal of a peaceful Outer Space'

The wording 'least likely to be true' in this question can be confusing. Another way of thinking of it is to look for the statement 'most likely to be false'.

It is possible to go through all the statements and check each one. A quicker way to narrow down your choice is to look at the wording. The word 'all' should stand out to you in the second statement. For this to be true, there should be not be any evidence of aggression by any nations. The last sentence talks about the deployment of weapons and testing of anti-satellite weapons. You can then quickly scan the text relating to the other statements to check that the 'could be true' and confirm your answer.

Question 2

Which of the following statements is true?

*   The United Nations was formed in 1927
*   Density of space at the Karman line is approximately one hydrogen atom per cubic meter
*   Under international law, Iran is permitted to send exploratory rockets in to Outer Space
*   Most stars reach temperatures of over one million Kelvin

Answer: 'Under international law, Iran is permitted to send exploratory rockets in to Outer Space'.

This is the only statement that can be confirmed in the passage. The Outer Space Treaty allows 'all states to explore outer space freely'. All the other statements could be true; however we can't definitively tell from the passage.

Question 3

Which of the following statements can be inferred from the passage?

*   The majority of nations believe that conflict is a distinct possibility in Outer Space
*   Attempts to prevent the deployment of weapons in Outer Space have been largely successful
*   Plasma is the hottest known substance in the Universe
*   Dark matter makes up the majority of mass in the Universe

Answer: 'The majority of nations believe that conflict is a distinct possibility in Outer Space.'

The fact that the United Nations has drafted treaties suggests that this is likely.

Question 4

Which of the following statements is false?

- Plasma is extremely hot despite being extremely low density in Outer Space
- Neutrinos are more common than hydrogen atoms in Outer Space
- There is an agreed clear definition of Outer Space
- The possibility of international agreement on matters relating to Outer Space is remote

Answer: 'The possibility of international agreement on matters relating to Outer Space is remote'

The passage gives a couple of examples of international treaties regarding Outer Space. As it has already happened, the possibility of international agreement can not be said to be 'remote', which implies 'highly unlikely'.

To confirm, look at the other statements briefly - statements 1 and 3 are confirmed in the passage. We can't tell whether neutrinos are more common or not than hydrogen atoms.

Verbal Reasoning Exercise

Try and do the following questions under 'timed conditions'. Allow yourself 1 minute for the instructions and then 10 minutes to answer the 5 questions that follow. answers are at the end of the section. As rough guide, we suggest allowing 40 seconds to scan the text and then 15-20 seconds to answer each question, checking back to the appropriate part of the text as required. The instructions are similar to those you will encounter in the real test.

Verbal Reasoning Instructions

Take 1 minute to read these instructions.

You will be presented with a passage to read. There will be four statements which are related to the passage. Using only the information in the passage, use logic to decide whether the statements are true, false or that you 'can't tell'.

True:
Using the information in the passage, you are able to say that you consider the statement to be true or that it follows logically from the passage.

False:
On the basis of the information contained in the passage, you can say that the statement is false.

Can't Tell:
You are unable to tell from the information in the passage whether the statement is true or false.

New question Type:

A new verbal reasoning type of question has been introduced. There will be four multiple-choice questions relating to a passage. You will be asked to draw conclusions regarding the passage.

You have 10 minutes to answer 20 items. Answer all the questions as there is no penalty for a wrong answer and blank questions will be marked incorrect.

10

Passage 1

Maverick's

Big wave surfing originated in Hawaii and became popular in California following the discovery of the waves at Maverick's point. These waves, approximately 2 miles from the nearest shore at Half-Moon Bay can routinely break over 25 feet and even up to 80 feet. An unusual rock formation underwater helps creates the waves.

Local boy Jeff Clark was the first to surf the big waves at Maverick's. In 1975, at the age of 17, he paddled out alone and caught a few left-breaking waves. For 15 years he surfed the waves alone, becoming part of surfing folklore. However, the wave did not get it's name from him. 'Maverick' was originally a dog who followed some surfers out nearby in the early 1960s. They deemed the huge waves unsuitable and named them after the dog, who had got the most out of the experience. Since 1990, the waves at Maverick's have been regularly surfed by surfers from all over the world. 1994 brought tragedy when the legendary Hawaiian big-wave surfer Mark Foo drowned surfing 18 foot waves. The spot gained a certain notoriety and sparked a debate about the safety of leashes in big waves. Foo may have drowned when he was unable to swim to the surface after his leash snagged on rocks. Nowadays, many big-wave surfers do not use leashes or have quick releases fitted to them for use in an emergency.

Big wave surfing contests have been held at Maverick's since 1999. The biggest waves are in the winter and the most common time for the competitions is March. Since 2010 the competition has been organised by the Half-Moon bay Surf Group.

Decide whether the following statements are 'true', 'false' or that you 'can't tell'

1. **Jeff Clark was born in 1958**   CT

2. **California is the best place in the world to surf big waves**   CT

3. **Surfing big waves in California is generally more dangerous than surfing big waves in Hawaii**   CT

4. **Jeff Clark is a well-known Californian surfer** T

(Passage adapted from Wikipedia, the free online encyclopaedia. http://en.wikipedia.org/wiki/Mavericks_(location))

11

Passage 2

The Diabetic Eye

When we look at something, light enters through the front of the eye and is focused by the lens onto the retina. The retina contains specialised cells known as 'rods' and 'cones' which are sensitive to light. Light is converted to electrical signals and these travel along the optic nerve to be interpreted by the brain. To work properly, the retina needs a good blood supply. Amongst other effects, diabetes can cause problems with these delicate retinal blood vessels.

In people with diabetes, glucose levels in the blood can be persistently higher than the rest of the population. Glucose can attach to proteins or lipids in the walls of vessels, a process known as glycosylation. The walls of the blood vessels then become prone to blockage and become leaky. Initially, the vessels only bulge slightly (micro aneurysms) and leak small amounts of blood or serum. Most diabetics are unaware of this process as it does not affect their visual capability and it is known as 'background retinopathy'. However, if the macula (the part of the retina where the lens focuses light) is affected then vision can be reduced.

As more vessels become blocked, whole areas of the retina become hypoxic, stimulating new growth of blood vessels to supply oxygen to the areas that are starved of it. These new blood vessels are often weak and on the surface of the retina. If they bleed, haemorrhages can totally obscure vision for short periods of time. Recurrent bleeds can lead to the development of scar tissue which can distort the shape of the retina, leading to an increased risk of detachment. This stage of retinopathy is known as 'proliferative diabetic retinopathy'. Fortunately, not all diabetics develop proliferative retinopathy. Laser treatments are available and with good control of blood sugar levels the risk is reduced.

Decide whether the following statements are 'true', 'false' or that you 'can't tell'

1. **Micro aneurysms are found only in the early stages of diabetic retinopathy** Ct

2. **The development of scar tissue does not lead to major eye problems** F

3. **The optic nerve is not affected by diabetes** CT

4. **Glycosylation is the root cause of diabetic retinal disease** T

Passage 3

The Ancient Olympic Games

At the height of their importance in the 6th and 5th Centuries BC, conflicts were postponed to allow the ancient Olympic games to proceed. Representatives of several different city-states and kingdoms came together to compete in events including athletics, combat and chariot-racing. Thought to have started in 776 BC the last ancient Games probably took place in 393 AD when emperor Theodosius I declared that all pagan cults and practices be eliminated. The Games were part of a cycle known as the Panhellenic Games and other events included the Pythian, Nemean and Isthmian Games. There was a religious significance to the ancient Games and ritual sacrifices were made to honour both Zeus and the mythical King Pelops.

In the legends of Ancient Greece, Heracles and his father Zeus were said to have started the Games. Heracles established them every 4 years and was said to have built the original Olympic stadium. On its completion he walked in a straight line for 200 steps, a distance that became known as a 'stadion'. The 'stadion event' became the equivalent of our 100 metre sprint and involved racing 192 yards around a wooden post and back. The first Olympic stadion champion is thought to be Coroebus, a cook from the city of Elis, who received an olive branch as a prize.

The ancient pentathlon involved jumping, discus, javelin, running and wrestling. Boxing and wrestling were popular, as was 'pankration', a blend of the two with almost no rules other than no biting or eye gouging. There were also musical and poetry contests in which women are thought to have taken part.

Decide whether the following statements are 'true', 'false' or that you 'can't tell'

1. **Ancient Greeks attached both religious and cultural importance to the Games**   T

2. **Women took part in all of the ancient Olympic events**   CT

3. **Pankration involved two fighters with almost no rules**   CT

4. **Emperor Theodosius is thought by historians to have believed the Olympic Games to be heretical**

(Passage adapted from Wikipedia, the free online encyclopaedia http://en.wikipedia.org/wiki/Ancient_Olympic_Games)

Passage 4

Whales

The Cetacean suborder *Mysticeti* includes the blue, humpback, bowhead and minke whales. These whales are filter feeders, eating small organisms which are removed from seawater by a comb-like structure inside the mouth known as a baleen. Their forelimbs are fins and their nasal openings form their blowhole. Like all mammals, whales breathe air, are warm blooded, produce milk for their young and have body hair.

The blue whale is the largest animal known to have existed and can grow to 30m in length and weigh 180 tonnes. There are at least 3 different subspecies found in all the different oceans of the world. They feed almost exclusively on zooplankton and an adult blue whale can eat up to 40 million krill, or 3600 Kg in a day. They hunt krill at depths of about 100m during the day and at the surface at night. Hunting dives can last for up to 30 minutes at a time. Blue whales themselves are so large they have virtually no natural predators, although up to a quarter of blue whales have scars from orca (killer whale) attacks.

The gestation period is 12 months and females give birth every two to three years to a calf that can weigh 3 tonnes. Sexual maturity is reached at about 7 years and total lifespan could be over 100 years, although no studies have been lengthy enough to ascertain this for certain.

In 2002, there were an estimated 8000 blue whales worldwide. Their numbers were decimated by commercial whaling in the 19th and early 20th centuries, reducing the population from an approximate 800,000 worldwide. Since the introduction of the whaling ban, best estimates show an increase of 7.3 % per year but numbers remain at under 1% of what they were pre-whaling.

Decide whether the following statements are 'true', 'false' or that you 'can't tell'

1. **Krill descend during the day and come to the surface at night**

2. **Krill are a type of zooplankton**

3. **The population of all types of whale (in the suborder Mysticeti) was reduced by whaling**

4. **Some types of mammal do not produce milk for their young**

(Passage adapted from wikipedia, the free online encyclopaedia http://en.wikipedia.org/wiki/Whales)

14

Passage 5

The Mayor of Casterbridge

Lucetta's reply was taken from her lips by an unexpected diversion. A bye-road on her right hand descended from the fields into the highway at the point where she stood, and down the track a bull was rambling uncertainly towards her and Elizabeth, who, facing the other way, did not observe him.

In the latter quarter of each year cattle were at once the mainstay and the terror of families about Casterbridge and its neighbourhood, where breeding was carried on with Abrahamic success. The head of stock driven into and out of the town at this season to be sold by the local auctioneer was very large; and all these horned beasts, in travelling to and fro, sent women and children to shelter as nothing else could do. In the main the animals would have walked along quietly enough; but the Casterbridge tradition was that to drive stock it was indispensable that hideous cries coupled with yahoo antics and gestures should be used, large sticks flourished, stray dogs called in, and in general everything was done that was likely to infuriate the viciously disposed and terrify the mild. Nothing was commoner than for a householder, on going out of his parlour, to find his hall or passage full of little children, nursemaids, aged women, or a ladies' school, who apologised for their presence by saying "A bull passing down street from sale."

Lucetta and Elizabeth regarded the animal in doubt, he meanwhile drawing vaguely towards them. It was a large specimen of the breed, in colour rich dun, though disfigured at present by splotches of mud about his seamy sides. His horns were thick and tipped with brass; his two nostrils like the Thames tunnel as seen in the perspective toys of yore. Between them, through the gristle of his nose, was a stout copper ring, welded on, and irremovable as Gurth's collar of brass. To the ring was attached an ash staff about a yard long, which the bull with the motions of his head flung about like a flail.

(Passage source: The Mayor of Casterbridge by Thomas Hardy)

Which of the following statements is true?

1. Lucetta is older than Elizabeth

2. There are many cattle in Casterbridge throughout the year

3. Householders are becoming annoyed with people sheltering in their halls from cattle

4. Large numbers of cattle are driven through Casterbridge every October

Which of the following statements is least likely to be true?

1. The bull has come from the field on Lucetta's right side

2. Most cattle in Casterbridge have their horns removed early in their lives

3. Some of the cattle are afraid of the people of Casterbridge

4. People in Casterbridge treat their animals with kindness and compassion

Which of the following statements is false?

1. Most cattle in Casterbridge are by nature placid

2. Lucetta is nervous of the bull approaching her

3. Bulls are not driven though the streets of Casterbridge

4. Small numbers of cattle are bred around Casterbridge

Which of the following statements can be inferred from the passage?

1. Elizabeth is in more danger than Lucetta

2. The bull is likely to have escaped from its owner

3. Wild bulls roamed the streets in 19th century England

4. The bull is enraged and has been rolling in the mud

Answers:

Passage 1:

1. Statement: Jeff Clark was born in 1958

Answer: Can't Say Although Jeff Clark was age 17 at some point in 1975, he could have been born in 1957, 1958 or 1959

2. Statement: California is the best place in the world to surf big waves

Answer: Can't say This may or may not be true. There is no explicit evidence in the passage to be able to answer this definitively. It is also likely to be a subjective judgement and answers would probably vary from surfer to surfer.

3. Statement: Surfing big waves in California is generally more dangerous than surfing big waves in Hawaii

Answer: Can't say Although a Hawaiian surfer drowned at Maverick's in California, this does not mean that it is 'generally more dangerous' to surf in California

4. Statement: Jeff Clark is a well-known Californian surfer

Answer: True Jeff Clark 'became part of surfing folklore' and was a 'local-boy' to Maverick's point in California. He is therefore a 'well-known Californian surfer'

Passage 2:

1. Micro aneurysms are found only in the early stages of diabetic retinopathy

Answer: Can't say Although this seems unlikely, there is nothing in the passage to indicate whether this is the case or not - we only know that they are found in the first stage of retinopathy, 'background retinopathy'.

2. The development of scar tissue does not lead to major eye problems

Answer: False We are told that scar tissue can distort the shape of the retina and lead to an increased risk of retinal detachment. These are major eye problems.

3. The optic nerve is not affected by diabetes

Answer: Can't say The article does not tell us how or whether the optic nerve is affected in diabetes, so we 'can't say'. In fact, glycosylation of nerves is a big problem in diabetes and is known as 'diabetic neuropathy'.

4. Glycosylation is the root cause of diabetic retinal disease

Answer: True The article explains that glycosylation leads to leaky and blocked blood vessels which lead to diabetic retinal disease (retinopathy)

Passage 3:

1. Ancient Greeks attached both religious and cultural importance to the Games

Answer: True According to the passage, ritual sacrifices were made and conflict was stopped to allow the Games to proceed.

2. Women took part in all of the ancient Olympic events

Answer: Can't say We are told they are thought to have taken part in musical and poetry events, but not whether or not they took part in other events

3. Pankration involved two fighters with almost no rules

Answer: Can't say We are not told how many fighters were involved in a pankration contest, although we are told there were almost no rules

4. Emperor Theodosius is thought by historians to have believed the Olympic Games to be heretical

Answer: True The Games are 'thought' to have ended in AD 393 when the 'Emperor declared all pagan cults and practices be eliminated', suggesting that historians believe he thought the Games were heretical

Passage 4:

1. Krill descend during the day and come to the surface at night

Answer: Can't say This is the pattern that blue whales hunt them in and seems likely. However, there could be other explanations for this pattern of behaviour by blue whales and we can't come to this conclusion with certainty.

2. Krill are a type of zooplankton

Answer: True The article states: 'They feed almost exclusively on zooplankton and eat up to 3600Kg of krill in a day'. 3600kg is not an insignificant amount and so it follows krill are a type of zooplankton.

3. The population of all types of whale (in the suborder Mysticeti) was reduced by whaling

Answer: Can't say There is no information about how the population of other types of whale was affected by hunting.

4. Some types of mammal do not produce milk for their young

Answer: False The article states that 'Like all mammals, whales... produce milk for their young'

Passage 5:

1. Large numbers of cattle are driven through Casterbridge every October

We can't tell how old either Lucetta or Elizabeth are. We are told there are many cattle in Casterbridge in the latter quarter of the year but don't know about the rest of the year. Although people apologise to householders for sheltering, we can't tell if householders are becoming annoyed by it. The last statement, that 'large numbers of cattle are driven through Casterbridge every October' is confirmed at the start of the second paragraph.

2. People in Casterbridge treat their animals with kindness and compassion

It is unlikely people in Casterbridge treat their animals with kindness and compassion. The evidence is in the way they herd their cattle with 'hideous cries, large stick and stray dogs, doing everything to infuriate'

3. Bulls are not driven though the streets of Casterbridge

Bulls are driven though Casterbridge - people apologise for their presence by saying "A bull passing down street from sale"

4. The bull is likely to have escaped from its owner

The bull is clearly not wild - it has a ring through its nose. The staff attached to the ring indicates it may have been being led somewhere and has now escaped. Although the bull is probably enraged as it is 'flinging its head about like a flail', we can't tell whether it has been rolling in the mud. There is no indication that Elizabeth is in more danger than Lucetta - although initially she had not seen the bull, later it is stated that 'they both regarded the animal in doubt'.

Verbal Reasoning Practice Questions

Allow yourself the following amount of time, depending on how many questions you want to do:

1 passage: 2 minutes
2 passages: 4 minutes
5 passages: 9 minutes 40 seconds
11 passages: 21 minutes

Passage 1: 3D Printing

3D printing, or 'additive manufacturing' is a process of making three-dimensional solid objects from a digital file. 3D printing is achieved using 'additive processes' where an object is created by laying down successive layers of material. It is distinct from traditional techniques which mostly rely on the removal of material by drilling and cutting and are known as 'subtractive processes'.

3D printing technology has been used in the varied fields of industrial design, architecture, engineering, aerospace and medicine and dentistry.

Computer-aided designs are transformed into thin, virtual, horizontal cross-sections. The machine then lays down successive layers of liquid, powder, or sheet material, and in this way builds up the model from the series of cross sections. These layers are joined together or fused automatically to create the final shape. The primary advantage to additive fabrication is its ability to create almost any shape or geometric feature.

The standard data interface between CAD software and the machines is the STL file format. An STL file approximates the shape of a part or assembly using triangular facets. Smaller facets produce a higher quality surface. VRML files are often used as input for 3D printing technologies that are able to print in full colour.

Construction of a model with contemporary methods can take from several hours to several days, depending on the method used and the size and complexity of the model. Additive systems can typically produce models in a few hours, although it can vary widely depending on the type of machine being used and the size and number of models being produced simultaneously.
Some techniques use two materials in the course of constructing parts. The first material is the part material and the second is the support material (to support overhanging features during construction). The support material is later removed by heat or dissolved away with a solvent or water.

Traditional injection moulding can be less expensive for manufacturing polymer products in high quantities, but additive fabrication can be faster and less expensive when producing relatively small quantities of parts. 3D printers give designers and concept development teams the ability to produce parts and concept models using a desktop size printer.

(Passage adapted from wikipedia, the free online encyclopaedia
http://en.wikipedia.org/wiki/3d_printing)

Decide whether the following statements are true, false or that you can't tell:

1. **3D printing is likely to take over from traditional methods of manufacturing in the future**

2. **3D printing is useful for producing prototype models**

3. **The most common way of 3D printing uses two materials**

4. **3D printing can produce any shape desired**

Passage 2: A Damning Report for US Food Chains

There is no such thing as a 'Kid's meal' without too many calories, a report by the Centre for Medical Health in the Public Interest has said. This report looked at the nutritional quality of children's meals in 19 major restaurant chains. 91 percent of 1,974 possible combinations of meal at the 19 chains exceed 430 calories (1/3 of the recommended calorific intake for children aged 4 - 8 per day, as recommended by the National Consortium for Medicine).

There may be some healthy choices on restaurant menus, but parents generally have to navigate a minefield of fat, salt and calories to find them. For example, Ben's Bar and Grill has 500 different possible combinations of kids' meals, but 90 percent of them are too high in calories. One example combination comprises of 2 fried chicken wings, French fries, ice-cream and a chocolate milkshake, totalling 1320 calories.

A spokeswoman for the report has been looking into the issue. In response, fast-food-chain Hungry Joe's recently released a statement saying the chain is "pleased to offer a wide variety of kids meals with healthier options and lower calories". Calls to other restaurant chains over the week have not been returned. Bob's Dairy, Jimmy's and Bushtucker weren't included in the report as they do not disclose nutritional information regarding their meals.

Decide whether the following statements are true, false or that you can't tell:

1. **Children in the United States consume in excess of the daily amount of calorific intake recommended by the National Consortium for Medicine**

2. **Hungry Joe's serves more healthy meals than the other restaurant chains in the survey**

3. **The milkshake at Ben's Bar and Grill is high in calories**

4. **The recommended calorific intake for a 6 year old is 1420 calories**

Passage 3: Big Brother is Watching You

Sociological experiments throughout time have demonstrated the startling way in which people adopt their behaviour when they are in the presence of a pair of eyes, even if they haven't consciously noticed that they are there. Not only real pairs of eyes, but even something as simple as a portrait on the wall, the Mona Lisa perhaps!

For example, consider the dictator game. In its most basic form there are two players. Player A (the dictator) is given a sum of money. Player A then gets to decide whether to share the money with the second player, player B, and also how much, if any, they wish to give. The dictator keeps whatever they do not give away. If this game is played anonymously, such as over the internet, so that neither Player A nor Player B can identify each other you probably won't be surprised to learn that most dictators don't share.

However, that isn't the most interesting aspect of the game! When two eyespots are included on the background computer screen the dictators are much more likely to share money. Moreover, in a more complicated version of the game including a picture of a robot with human-like eyes again players are more likely to give money.

Another experiment was conducted in the North of England. Scientists asked people to pay for coffee in their staff room by putting money into a box (an honesty box). They put a picture of a pair of eyes above the box in some weeks and a bunch of flowers in others. In the weeks with the pair of eyes, people paid more often!

This raises some interesting questions about our social behaviour in a wider context. Our cities are covered with images of faces, in what way does this influence our behaviour? It may be that some images could reduce crime or reduce anti-social behaviour. It might be time to start using these in addition to, or instead of, expensive CCTV cameras. After all, big brother is watching you.

Decide whether the following statements are true, false or that you can't tell:

1. **The article gives us good evidence that most people are dishonest when they think they are not being watched**

2. **The dictator game provides good evidence that people are more likely to share if they feel they are being watched**

3. **Visual images could possibly be used to influence the behaviour of people**

4. **Anti-social behaviour can be reduced by putting pictures of eyes on walls**

Passage 4: Trial at The Hague

A judge at the Special Court for Sierra Leone has found Charles Taylor guilty of aiding and abetting war crimes during the civil war in Sierra Leone. Taylor has been on trial for five years at the Hague, accused of backing the rebels of the Revolutionary United Front who killed tens of thousands between 1991 and 2002. Taylor was the president of neighbouring Liberia between 1997 and 2003. He went in to exile in Nigeria for a short while before being arrested in 2006 and sent for trial.

'This is a historic decision' stated Jordi Hulsker of Human Rights Action in Africa. 'A message has been sent to all high-ranking state officials around the world. There will be repercussions if you do not respect human rights. If you commit atrocities you will be held accountable.'

The judge said ' Taylor sold diamonds and bought weapons on behalf of the RUF rebels. He knew they were committing crimes. It is beyond reasonable doubt that the accused is criminally responsible.'

Mr Taylor will be sentenced later in the month and is expected to serve his sentence in a British prison. The Dutch government only agreed to host the trial if any jail term was served in a different country.

Decide whether the following statements are true, false or that you can't tell:

1. **Charles Taylor committed atrocities in Sierra Leone**

2. **Jordi Hulsker believes Charles Taylor committed atrocities**

3. **The RUF were responsible for the deaths of thousands of people**

4. **The judge was from Holland**

Passage 5: The Interpretation of Dreams

Read the following passage written by Sigmund Freud:

"I have isolated from the psychology of the dream the problem as to whether and to what extent the moral dispositions and feelings of waking life extend into dream-life. The same contradictions which we were surprised to observe in the descriptions by various authors of all the other psychic activities will surprise us again here. Some writers flatly assert that dreams know nothing of moral obligations; others as decidedly declare that the moral nature of man persists even in his dream-life.

Our ordinary experience of dreams seems to confirm beyond all doubt the correctness of the first assertion. As Jessen points out, one does not become better or more virtuous during sleep; on the contrary, it seems that conscience is silent in our dreams, inasmuch as one feels no compassion and can commit the worst crimes, such as theft, murder, and homicide, with perfect indifference and without subsequent remorse.

Radestock says: "It is to be noted that in dreams associations are effected and ideas combined without being in any way influenced by reflection, reason, aesthetic taste, and moral judgment; the judgment is extremely weak, and ethical indifference reigns supreme."

Volkelt expresses himself as follows: "As everyone knows, dreams are especially unbridled in sexual matters. Just as the dreamer himself is shameless in the extreme, and wholly lacking in moral feeling and judgment, so likewise does he see others, even the most respected persons, doing things which, even in his thoughts, he would blush to associate with them in his waking state."

Schopenhauer believes, in sharp contradiction to those mentioned above, that in dreams every man acts and talks in complete accordance with his character. Fischer also maintains that subjective feelings and desires, or affects and passions, manifest themselves in the wilfulness of the dream-life, and that the moral characteristics of a man are mirrored in his dreams."

Decide whether the following statements are true, false or that you can't tell:

1. **Jessen and Radestock agree that moral judgement is suspended in dreams**

2. **Freud believes, in contrast to Schopenhauer, that our dreams are not influenced by morality or ethical judgement**

3. **Radestock has had immoral dreams**

4. **Dreams usually involve morally questionable behaviour**

Passage 6: Dutch Elm Disease

In 1910, Dutch Elm Disease was discovered in north-west Europe. It was identified in Holland and found to be caused by a fungus, spread by the elm bark beetle. Dr Tom Peace began monitoring its rapid spread into Britain in the late 1920s and monitored the first epidemic which finished in the 1940s. By this time 10-40% of elms in different European countries had been lost. However, with the disease waning, Peace felt able to state that 'unless the trend of the disease completely changes, the disaster that once seemed inevitable will not come to pass'. Unfortunately, there was a change and in the late 1960s a second more destructive period of loss began.

The second outbreak of Dutch Elm Disease was caused by a different, more aggressive fungus and imported to Britain on infested elm logs from North America. Within the decade, an estimated 20 million of a total of 30 million UK elms were dead. The number continues to decline and the disease is gradually spreading northwards. Inverness was reached in 2006.

Elms used to be a familiar sight in the UK. Now, mature elms are only found in isolated pockets. The largest concentration is in Brighton, where in 2005 there were 15,000 elms surviving. Around the country, elms survive in low-cut hedges. Their roots are not killed and still send up shoots, although these usually succumb to the disease by the time they reach 5m.

Amsterdam has 75,000 elms lining its canals. Many of these were bred to be resistant to the fungus by introducing genes from the Himalayan elm.

Decide whether the following statements are true, false or that you can't tell:

1. **None of the elms found in the UK are resistant to Dutch Elm Disease**

2. **2/3 of UK elms were lost by the end of the 1970s**

3. **In 1950 Dr Peace felt that the loss of most elms was inevitable in the UK**

4. **Himalayan elms are not killed by the fungus that causes Dutch Elm disease**

Passage 7: Health Policy

Richard Paterson, the health secretary, has decided that NHS staff in poorer parts of the country should be paid less than their counterparts in richer areas. The changes would mean that cleaners, cooks, porters and clinical staff including nurses and midwives would earn less in the North of England than the South. There would be only one group exempted: the highest-paid managers who are in the process of delivering the controversial NHS reforms would not be included in the new regional pay-scale.

A Liberal Democrat spokesman said: 'Not satisfied with increasing the divisions between the north and the south, these proposals will also increase the divisions between the well-paid and the rest. This is a classic example of Paterson's ability to alienate the people he needs to rely on the most - NHS staff'.

The proposal may well become reality, as Paterson needs to push through measures to reduce the overall cost of running the NHS. The chancellor has decreed that the public sector should mimic the private sector and be more reflective of local economic conditions. He has given his backing to Paterson. Unions have responded angrily, saying that women will be particularly hit and that the government is 'out of touch with the public'. With opposition mounting it looks as though Paterson's in for a long fight, but with powerful backing he may well win.

Decide whether the following statements are true, false or that you can't tell:

1. The unions think that Richard Paterson is 'out of touch'

2. Under the new proposal, doctors in London would earn more than doctors in less well-off areas

3. The liberal democrats are part of a coalition government

4. This is the first time Paterson has caused controversy as health secretary

Passage 8: Never forget To Floss

A study was recently published in the Journal of Periodontology (JOP), the official publication of the American Academy of Periodontology, which highlights the importance of flossing as part of routine oral care. In fact, regular flossing can actually help reduce the amount of gum-disease-causing bacteria in the mouth, thus improving the overall health of teeth and gums.

The study looked at 51 sets of twins between the ages of 12 and 21. One set was randomly assigned to a 14 day regimen of manual brushing with toothpaste, whilst the comparable twin in the other set was asked to floss and brush. At the end of the trial samples were taken from either set and tested for bacteria commonly associated with periodontal disease. The results concluded that flossing in addition to brushing significantly lowers the levels of periodontal disease causing bacteria in the mouth compared with brushing alone.

The twin experimental model was specifically used to help control for genetic and environmental factors that can confound the results seen in treatment studies. Twins are likely to share the same life-style practices, dietary habits and, of course, genetics, which helps to lessen the impact of these external factors on the results. Essentially the addition of flossing as a treatment was isolated by the study.

"As a practising periodontologist, I often tell my patients to include flossing as part of their routine. Patients seem to think that it can't make that much difference, but the results of this study confirm the old adage that flossing is an important part of your dental care routing." Says Dr Jane Kelly.

Decide whether the following statements are true, false or that you can't tell:

1. **Most people in the United States underestimate the importance of flossing as part of their dental care routine**

2. **The results of the study would be less useful if twins were not used as test-subjects**

3. **Brushing alone does not reduce levels of periodontal disease-causing bacteria**

4. **Genetic factors rarely confound treatment studies**

Passage 9: Snake Fangs

Snake fangs are one of nature's most complex bioweapons and the question of how they evolved has perplexed scientists for many years. It now seems that the puzzle of the origin of snake fangs and their associated venom glands has been solved - they may have evolved as a result of a simple embryological change.

Both cobras and vipers have large, hollow fangs at the front of their mouths and use venom, a modified form of saliva, to immobilise or kill their prey. Other types of snakes have fangs at the back of the mouth or even no fangs at all. Vipers and cobras, the most venomous types of snakes, are only very distantly related. This would suggest that their fangs have evolved independently, which seems counter-intuitive. Why would such a sophisticated apparatus have evolved twice? Professor Alberto Vonk has been looking at whether snakes with front fangs and snakes with front and rear fangs share the same evolutional origin.

Vonk and his colleagues analysed the fang development in 96 embryos from eight living species and have shown that both front and rear fangs develop from separate teeth-forming tissue at the back of the upper jaw. For all front-fanged venomous snake species, the front fangs are displaced by rapid growth of embryonic upper jaws during development. In snakes with rear fangs, they stay where they are formed.

The separate development of the rear part of the tissue says Vonk, may have played an important role in snake's ability to diverge into the 3,000 species found in the world today.

"It sheds light on one of those nagging questions in herpetology - how did a diversity of fang types among snakes evolve?" said David Kizirian, a herpetologist at the American Museum of Natural History in New York.

Decide whether the following statements are true, false or that you can't tell:

1. **Professor Alberto Vonk is a leading herpetologist**

2. **Fangs at the front of the mouth tend to be more venomous than fangs at the back**

3. **Cobras and vipers are the only types of snake with fangs at the front of their mouths**

4. **All types of viper are venomous**

Passage 10: Twenty Thousand Leagues Under the Sea by Jules Verne, Chapter XIV

The next day was the 9th of November. I awoke after a long sleep of twelve hours. Conseil came, according to custom, to know 'how I passed the night,' and to offer his services. He had left his friend the Canadian sleeping like a man who had never done anything else all his life. I let the worthy fellow chatter as he pleased, without caring to answer him. I was preoccupied by the absence of the Captain during our sitting of the day before, and hoping to see him today.

As soon as I was dressed I went in to the saloon. It was deserted. I plunged into the study of the shell treasures hidden behind the glasses.

The whole day passed without my being honoured by a visit from Captain Nemo. The panes of the saloon did not open. Perhaps they did not wish us to tire of these beautiful things.

The course of the Nautilus was ENE, her speed twelve knots, the depth below the surface between twenty-five and thirty fathoms.

The next day, the 10th of November, the same desertion, the same solitude. I did not see one of the ship's crew: Ned and Conseil spent the greater part of the day with me. They were astonished at the puzzling absence of the Captain. Was this singular man ill? Had he altered his intentions with regard to us?

After all, as Conseil said, we enjoyed perfect liberty, we were delicately and abundantly fed. Our host kept to his terms of the treaty. We could not complain, and, indeed, the singularity of our fate reserved such wonderful compensation for us that we had no right to accuse it as yet.

(Source: http://www.gutenberg.org/files/164/164-h/164-h.htm#chap14)

Decide whether the following statements are true, false or that you can't tell:

1. **Conseil is employed by Captain Nemo**

2. **The Nautilus is a submarine**

3. **The Captain is making sure that the narrator is well looked after**

4. **The Captain has been too busy to see the Narrator, Ned and Conseil**

Passage 11: The Adventure of the Copper Beeches by Sir Arthur Conan Doyle

As he spoke the door opened and a young lady entered the room. She was plainly but neatly dressed, with a bright, quick face, freckled like a plover's egg, and with the brisk manner of a woman who has had her own way to make in the world.

"You will excuse my troubling you, I am sure," said she, as my companion rose to greet her, "but I have had a very strange experience, and as I have no parents or relations of any sort from whom I could ask advice, I thought that perhaps you would be kind enough to tell me what I should do."

"Pray take a seat, Miss Hunter. I shall be happy to do anything that I can to serve you."

I could see that Holmes was favourably impressed by the manner and speech of his new client. He looked her over in his searching fashion, and then composed himself, with his lids drooping and his fingertips together, to listen to her story.

"I have been a governess for five years," said she, "in the family of Colonel Spence Munro, but two months ago the Colonel received an appointment at Halifax, in Nova Scotia, and took his children over to America with him, so that I found myself without a situation. I advertised, and I answered advertisements but without success. At last the little money which I had saved began to run short, and I was at my wit's end as to what I should do."

"There is a well-known agency for governesses in the West End called Westaway's, and there I used to call about once a week in order to see whether anything had turned up which might suit me. Westaway was the name of the founder of the business, but it is really managed by Miss Stoper. She sits in her own little office, and the ladies who are seeking employment wait in an anteroom, and are then shown in one by one, when she consults her ledgers and sees whether she has anything which would suit them'"

"Well, when I called last week I was shown into the little office as usual, but I found that Miss Stoper was not alone. A prodigiously stout man with a very smiling face and a great heavy chin which rolled down in fold upon fold over his throat sat at her elbow with a pair of glasses on his nose, looking very earnestly at the ladies who entered. As I came in he gave quite a jump in his chair and turned quickly to Miss Stoper. That one may do, he said."
(Source: http://etext.lib.virginia.edu/toc/modeng/public/DoyBeec.html)

1. Which of the following statements is most likely to be true?

a) Miss Hunter is going to work for Miss Stoper
b) The stout man is looking for a woman exactly like Miss Hunter
c) Miss Hunter wanted to go to Halifax with the Colonel and his family
d) Miss Stoper owns the Westaway business
e) Miss Hunter considers Sherlock Holmes to be trustworthy

2. Which of the following statements can be inferred from the passage?

a) Governesses were relatively well paid in Victorian times
b) Colonel Spence Munro was a very well paid man
c) Many women wished to work as governesses at that time
d) It was a rare thing to be obese in the Victorian era
e) Miss Stoper was fond of Miss Hunter

3. Which of the following statements is false?

a) Colonel Spence Munro is an American
b) Sherlock Holmes would like to help Miss Hunter
c) The stout man has bad intentions towards Miss Hunter
d) Sherlock Holmes is tired
e) Colonel Spence Munro has one child

4. Which of the following statements is least likely to be true?

a) The obese man wishes to employ a young woman
b) Miss Hunter was not an effective governess
c) Miss Hunter did not have an easy start to life
d) Sherlock Holmes likes Miss Hunter
e) Miss Hunter takes care over her appearance

Passage 12: The War On Smoking

The war on smoking, especially following recent anti-smoking laws in some European countries, is being won in the west. However, worldwide, the death toll from smoking-related illnesses is still increasing as poorer countries are stepping in to take on the burden.

Tobacco is the single greatest cause of preventable death globally. Smoking increases the risk of heart attacks, strokes, chronic obstructive pulmonary disease and lung, mouth and pancreatic cancer. Peripheral vascular disease and hypertension are also associated. In underdeveloped countries, cigarettes tend to have a higher tar content and are less likely to be filtered, potentially increasing vulnerability to tobacco-related diseases in these countries. Second-hand smoke has also been shown to cause adverse health effects in people of all ages.

Some authors have claimed that by 2025 100 million deaths will have been caused by smoking worldwide. Research from the University of Oxford suggests that annual tobacco related deaths worldwide had reached 3.5 million in 1997. Longer life expectancies and bigger populations, together with the increasing trend in female smoking is also likely to increase this figure in the future.

China is a prime example of the situation. The tobacco epidemic has developed faster than any previous forecasts. New studies estimated that China has more tobacco deaths than any other country. Moreover, many of the smoking-related illnesses in China follow a different pattern to those typical in the west; with nearly half of all deaths caused by chronic obstructive pulmonary disease compared with just 15% in developed countries.

Decide whether the following statements are true, false or that you can't tell:

1. **The previous forecast of a slow rate of uptake in smoking within China has now been shown to be incorrect**

2. **Chronic obstructive pulmonary disease is more common in China than in developed countries**

3. **Lung cancer is usually caused by smoking**

4. **Smoking-related deaths are reducing in some European countries but increasing in developing countries**

Passage 13: Transistor Radios

A transistor radio is a small portable radio receiver that uses transistor-based circuitry. Following their development in 1954 they became the most popular electronic communication device in history, with billions manufactured during the 1960s and 1970s. Their small size sparked a change in popular music listening habits, allowing people to listen to music anywhere they went. In the 1970s their popularity declined as other portable media players such as boom boxes and portable cassette players took over.

The use of transistors instead of vacuum tubes as amplifier elements meant that the device was much smaller, required far less power to operate than a tube radio and was more shock-resistant. Transistors are current amplifiers, while tubes are voltage amplifiers. This allows 'instant on' operation since there are no filaments to heat up.

Some estimates suggest that there are at least seven billion transistor radios in existence, almost all tunable to the common AM band and many also tunable to the FM band. Most operate on battery power and are small and cheap. Virtually all commercial broadcast receivers are now transistor based.

In the 1950s and 1960s, the popularity of transistor radios was also benefited from social forces. There were a large number of young people around as a result of the post World War 2 baby boom; it was a period of increased prosperity and an increased disposable income and rock 'n' roll music was becoming increasingly popular.

Decide whether the following statements are true, false or that you can't tell:

1. **Transistor radios are the most popular communication device in history**

2. **Most commercial broadcast receivers make use of voltage amplification**

3. **The popularity of transistor radios was mostly due to increasing prosperity following World War 2**

4. **In the 1970s boom boxes were more popular than transistor radios**

(Passage adapted from wikipedia, the online free encyclopaedia http://en.wikipedia.org/wiki/Transistor_radio)

Passage 14: A Mayor's Vision

The new mayor of Karachi, Syed Mustafa Kamal, only 36 years old, has a vision for the future. He wants his city, a sprawling metropolis by the sea, to become world class. He has sworn his city will rival Dubai within five years and he's already made some progress!

He has begun by building a 47-storey Technology tower complete with a 10,000 seat call centre. This is one of the biggest in Asia. In order to ease congestion he has completed six under and over-passes together with a signal-free crosstown corridor. However, many see him as out of touch, with more than half of the 16 million population living in squatter settlements and shanty towns. Only around half of the city's daily water needs are met and power outages are commonplace. These problems perpetuate the ills of crime, congestion, political volatility and, recently, have led to terrorism.

Six bombs were detonated on July 20th across the city in short succession. A suicide bomber followed in October at the welcome-home rally for former Prime Minister Benazir Bhutto, killing 141. Kamal remains confident, stating emphatically "It can be done. It will be done. In five years time, I can turn this city around."

The problem is, he doesn't have control and nor does anyone else. Karachi is composed of 18 towns and 6 cantonments. A local board runs each cantonment and charges fees and makes plans as it deems appropriate. None of these boards are answerable to the city government. This administrative structure is a legacy of the previous military system inherited from the British.

Decide whether the following statements are true, false or that you can't tell:

1. **Poverty and lack of basic amenities is inciting acts of terrorism within Karachi**

2. **Syed Mustafa Kamal is Karachi's youngest ever Mayor**

3. **Syed Mustafa Kamal believes dealing with congestion is important to the successful creation of a world class metropolis**

4. **The Mayor of Karachi is out of touch with the local population**

Passage 15: Alcohol-Related Illness

Alcohol accounts for 6% of all hospital admissions in the UK. This figure, recently released by the Department of Health, shows that 811,443 people were admitted during the year 2006 - 2007 for alcohol-related reasons. This is 71% higher than the figure published in 2002 - 2003.

The reason for this increase is likely to be multifactorial. An important point to consider is that the definition of alcohol-related illness is wider and encompasses a greater number of conditions than that previously used in other reports.

The cost of the problem is colossal, with some estimates as high as £20 billion per annum - affecting nearly 8.2 million adults. Alcoholic liver disease, itself, is at its all time highest level in England - with alcohol now reaching the 3rd leading cause of ill health after tobacco and high blood pressure.

These figures have prompted the government to look more closely at the issue. In the near future UK alcohol manufacturers could be forced to provide similar warnings on alcoholic drinks bottles as those currently required on cigarette and tobacco packets. In the light of these recent statistics this would make logical sense. However, similar strategies in the US have failed to produce significant results.

Decide whether the following statements are true, false or that you can't tell:

1. **According to the department of health, 474,528 people were admitted during the year 2002 - 2003 for alcohol related reasons**

2. **Using the same criteria for 'alcohol-related-illnesses' across study years would lower the observed increase in alcohol-related hospital admissions on previous years**

3. **Rates of alcoholic liver disease are higher in England than in other parts of the UK**

4. **Forcing alcohol manufacturers to put warnings on their bottles is likely to reduce alcoholic liver disease**

(Passage adapted from wikipedia, the free online encyclopaedia
http://en.wikipedia.org/wiki/Alcohol_Related_Illness)

Passage 16: Black Holes

A black hole is a region of space-time from which nothing can escape. The theory of general relativity predicts that a sufficiently compact mass will deform space-time to form a black hole. Around a black hole there is a mathematically defined surface called an event horizon that marks the point of no return.

Objects whose gravity field is too strong for light to escape were first considered in the 18th Century by John Michell and Pierre Simon Laplace. Long considered a mathematical curiosity, it was during the 1960s that theoretical work showed black holes were a generic prediction of general relativity. The discovery of neutron stars sparked interest in gravitationally collapsed compact objects as a possible astrophysical reality.

Black holes of stellar masses are expected to form when very massive stars collapse at the end of their lifecycle. After a black hole has formed it can continue to grow by absorbing mass from its surroundings. Supermassive black holes of millions of solar masses may form and there is general consensus that these exist at the centre of most galaxies.

Decide whether the following statements are true, false or that you can't tell:

1. **It is impossible to escape from a black hole**

2. **The theory of general relativity is used to predict the existence of the 'event horizon'**

3. **Black holes commonly form when very massive stars collapse**

4. **Blue light is affected by gravity**

(Passage adapted from wikipedia, the free online encyclopaedia
http://en.wikipedia.org/wiki/Black_holes)

Passage 17: Glacier Retreat

The retreat of glaciers has been well-documented over the last century and seems to be accelerating. Over the last 40 years, glaciers in the French alps have lost a quarter of their area. New data has shown that since the late 1960s the area covered by ice in the Mont Blanc range has shrunk from 375 sq. km to 275 sq. km. The research was carried out by the University of Savoie and presented at the annual meeting of the American Geophysical Union.

The Mont Blanc massif was not the only region looked at. 600 glaciers in the Alps were studied in total, including areas to the south such as the Ecrins massif. Maps, satellite data and aerial photographs were used and the team sent field-workers to manually inspect some of the areas to check their methods were correct.

'We need to inspect some of the glaciers as there can be a problem with debris on the glacier obscuring some of the ice.' said a member of the team. 'Shadows can also cause difficulties when inspecting a satellite image, leading to incorrect data.'

A striking is result is the higher rate of retreat in the South of France. This may be due to the lower elevation of the mountains and the different climate. Less cloud and precipitation mean the glaciers are exposed to more sun and have less chance to build back up again in the winter.

At current rate of loss, there are likely to be very few Alpine glaciers by 2100. Glaciers will gradually become smaller and thinner and survive only in higher, colder areas.

Decide whether the following statements are true, false or that you can't tell:

1. **The team took careful measures to ensure that their data was correct**

2. **Glaciers have only been retreating for the last 40 years**

3. **Glaciers in the Ecrins massif are retreating quicker than those in the Mont Blanc massif**

4. **Glaciers all over the world are in retreat**

Passage 18: Hardangervidda

The Hardangervidda is a mountain plateau in western Norway. It is the largest plateau in Europe, with a cold alpine climate and contains one of Norway's largest glaciers. Much of the plateau is protected as part of the Hardangervidda National Park, which extends in to the counties of Buskerud, Hordaland and Telemark.

The plateau is a peneplain, or an 'eroded plain', and is the remnants of mountains that have been worn down by glaciers over millions of years. Most of the bedrock is from the Precambrian and Cambro-Silurian periods. Now, the landscape consists of barren, treeless moorland containing numerous pools, rivers and lakes. It is wetter on the west side, which is less vegetated due to large expanses of bare rock. The highest point is Sandfloeggi which reaches 1721m up.

The plateau is above the treeline and many arctic animals and plants are found here that are usually found further north. Reindeer herds cross the plateau, wintering on the east side and breeding on the west. About 8000 years ago when the climate was warmer, large parts of the plateau were wooded and pine logs can be found preserved in bogs well above today's treeline.

The National Park was formed in 1981 and is Norway's largest at 1321 square miles, encompassing most of the plateau and entirely above 1000m. There is a comprehensive system of huts and paths across the plateau and people use the area for hiking, climbing and fishing in the summer. In the winter cross-country skiing and kite-skiing are popular.

Decide whether the following statements are true, false or that you can't tell:

1. **Cross-country skiing takes place only in the winter on the Hardangervidda plateau**

2. **Part of the plateau is within the county of Hordaland**

3. **The treeline is below 1000m in this part of Norway**

4. **Most rivers on the plateau flow east to west**

(Passage adapted from wikipedia, the free online encyclopaedia
http://en.wikipedia.org/wiki/Hardangervidda)

Passage 19: It's Still Wine

The price of oil has reached record highs. This has spurred a renewed interest in ways to cut our dependence on oil and our part in preserving the environment. One important such area is recycling with many households now participating on a regular basis.

You may, therefore, be surprised to learn that the wine bottle is of greater detriment to the environment than its plastic counterpart! Weighing in at around 400 grams, it is typically 8 times heavier than a plastic equivalent, requires more energy to transport and therefore contributes to greater greenhouse gas emissions.

Many reputable French Chateaus have already succeeded in making the switch to the screw-cap and there is now hope of the same for the plastic bottle. Many wine connoisseurs throw their arms up in abhorrence at the very notion of drinking wine that comes in a plastic bottle, but change is already occurring.

One such producer, Arniston Bay from South Africa has even begun to experiment with plastic pouches. These are some one-twentieth of the weight of a glass counterpart. Such packaging is substantially out of favour in South Africa, where papsaks (foil bags containing wine) were banned - purportedly responsible for worsening alcoholism and social disruption within the country. In Britain, however, things may be significantly different...

Decide whether the following statements are true, false or that you can't tell:

1. **The transportation costs for a 'plastic pouch' are even less than those for a plastic bottle**

2. **England is likely to have a more relaxed approach to the use of plastic bottles for packaging wine than South Africa**

3. **The process of production of glass wine bottles is worse for the environment than production of plastic wine pouches**

4. **Wine from a plastic bottle tastes different to wine from a glass bottle**

Passage 20: Neurobiology – Hearing Movement!

The phenomenon of synaesthesia applies to those individuals who perceive the world in a very different way to the rest of us. In these individuals, their senses are cross-activated, that is, some synaesthetes perceive days of the week as possessing personalities, or, as we shall see, images as having sounds!

Recently, a research group at the California Institute of Technology has discovered synaesthetes who hear sounds (e.g. beeping, whirring or tapping) when they see things move or flash. Apparently, this phenomenon may not be as unusual as we think! The phenomenon was discovered purely by chance. Whilst running an experiment, one of the researchers happened to come across a group of students, one of which claimed to hear something whilst watching a movie of radially expanding dots. On further questioning it had all the hallmarks of an auditory synaesthesia. She then ran a series of further experiments and managed to identify a further four people all exhibiting the same trait.

Two other researchers, Saenz and Koch, found that these four synaesthetes outperformed a group of non-synaesthetes on a rhythmic pattern identification exercise. Normally these patterns are easier to identify if they are encoded in beeps rather than flashes, but the synaesthetes actually hear a beep when they see the flashes and so were able to outperform non-synaesthetes when tested with flash patterns alone.

Saenz and Koch suspect that up to 1% of the population may experience auditory synaesthesia. Very little is known about this phenomenon or how the auditory and visual systems within the brain work together. Understanding this interaction will help us to probe deeper into understanding the workings of our brains.

Decide whether the following statements are true, false or that you can't tell:

1. **The perception of letters or numbers as having a colour is an example of a synaesthesia**

2. **Individuals with synaesthesia outperform normal individuals on visual rhythmic pattern identification exercises such as that used in the study**

3. **Auditory synaesthetes are probably better at identifying visible rhythmic patterns than non-synaesthetes**

4. **Auditory synaesthesia is the most common type of synaesthesia**

Passage 21: 20 000 Leagues Under the Sea, by Jules Verne, Chapter XXX

The Mediterranean, the blue sea par excellence, "the great sea" of the Hebrews, "the sea" of the Greeks, the "mare nostrum" of the Romans, bordered by orange-trees, aloes, cacti, and sea-pines; embalmed with the perfume of the myrtle, surrounded by rude mountains, saturated with pure and transparent air, but incessantly worked by underground fires; a perfect battlefield in which Neptune and Pluto still dispute the empire of the world!

It is upon these banks, and on these waters, says Michelet, that man is renewed in one of the most powerful climates of the globe. But, beautiful as it was, I could only take a rapid glance at the basin whose superficial area is two million of square yards. Even Captain Nemo's knowledge was lost to me, for this puzzling person did not appear once during our passage at full speed. I estimated the course which the Nautilus took under the waves of the sea at about six hundred leagues, and it was accomplished in forty-eight hours. Starting on the morning of the 16th of February from the shores of Greece, we had crossed the Straits of Gibraltar by sunrise on the 18th.

It was plain to me that this Mediterranean, enclosed in the midst of those countries which he wished to avoid, was distasteful to Captain Nemo. Those waves and those breezes brought back too many remembrances, if not too many regrets. Here he had no longer that independence and that liberty of gait which he had when in the open seas, and his Nautilus felt itself cramped between the close shores of Africa and Europe.

Our speed was now twenty-five miles an hour. It may be well understood that Ned Land, to his great disgust, was obliged to renounce his intended flight. He could not launch the pinnace, going at the rate of twelve or thirteen yards every second. To quit the Nautilus under such conditions would be as bad as jumping from a train going at full speed--an imprudent thing, to say the least of it. Besides, our vessel only mounted to the surface of the waves at night to renew its stock of air; it was steered entirely by the compass and the log.

(Source: http://www.gutenberg.org/ebooks/2488)

1. Which of the following statements is most likely to be false?

a) The Mediterranean was the largest sea known to the Hebrews
b) Michelet loves the Mediterranean
c) Captain Nemo has previously travelled in the Mediterranean
d) The Nautilus made two brief stops on its passage through the Mediterranean
e) At night, the Nautilus mostly travelled beneath the surface

2. Which of the following is most likely to be true?

a) The Captain is pleased to be in the Mediterranean sea
b) The Captain is pushing the Nautilus to it's top speed
c) Ned Land is trying to escape the Nautilus
d) Michelet was a famous French travel writer
e) There was calm weather on the surface of the Mediterranean as the Nautilus passed through.

3. Which of the following statements is false?

a) A pinnace is a type of boat
b) The Nautilus usually travels at a depth of 100 leagues
c) There are active volcanoes beneath the Mediterranean
d) Compasses work well beneath the sea
e) It took less than 72 hours to travel from Greece to the Straits of Gibraltar

4. Which of the following statements is true?

a) Cacti grow in all of the countries bordering the Mediterranean
b) Captain Nemo has extensive knowledge of the Mediterranean
c) It is not far from North Africa to Europe
d) Neptune and Pluto are Roman gods
e) There is enough air on the Nautilus for the crew for at least 8 hours

Passage 22: Chapter 2, The Mayor of Casterbridge by Thomas Hardy

The morning sun was streaming through the crevices of the canvas when the man awoke. A warm glow pervaded the whole atmosphere of the marquee, and a single big blue fly buzzed musically round and round it. Besides the buzz of the fly there was not a sound. He looked about - at the benches - at the table supported by trestles - at his basket of tools - at the stove where the furmity had been boiled - at the empty basins - at some shed grains of wheat - at the corks which dotted the grassy floor. Among the odds and ends he discerned a little shining object, and picked it up. It was his wife's ring.

A confused picture of the events of the previous evening seemed to come back to him, and he thrust his hand into his breast-pocket. A rustling revealed the sailor's bank-notes thrust carelessly in.

This second verification of his dim memories was enough; he knew now they were not dreams. He remained seated, looking on the ground for some time. "I must get out of this as soon as I can," he said deliberately at last, with the air of one who could not catch his thoughts without pronouncing them. "She's gone - to be sure she is - gone with that sailor who bought her, and little Elizabeth-Jane. We walked here, and I had the furmity, and rum in it - and sold her. Yes, that's what's happened and here am I. Now, what am I to do - am I sober enough to walk, I wonder?" He stood up, found that he was in fairly good condition for progress, unencumbered. Next he shouldered his tool basket, and found he could carry it. Then lifting the tent door he emerged into the open air.

Here the man looked around with gloomy curiosity. The freshness of the September morning inspired and braced him as he stood. He and his family had been weary when they arrived the night before, and they had observed but little of the place; so that he now beheld it as a new thing. It exhibited itself as the top of an open down, bounded on one extreme by a plantation, and approached by a winding road. At the bottom stood the village that lent its name to the upland and the annual fair that was held thereon. The views stretched downward into valleys, and onward to other uplands, dotted with barrows, and trenched with the remains of prehistoric forts.

NB: 'Furmity' refers to a dish of wheat boiled with milk and spices.

(Source: http://www.online-literature.com/hardy/casterbridge/)

1. Which of the following statements is most likely to be true?

a) The man remembers nothing of the previous night.
b) Elizabeth-Jane is likely to be the man's daughter
c) The man was happily married
d) Furmity is usually mixed with rum
e) It is likely that the man will find his wife again

2. Which of the following statements is false?

a) The passage is set on a fine September's day
b) The man is still drunk
c) His wife's ring was very expensive
d) The shed he has woken up in is set on top of a hill
e) The man sold his wife for a pittance

3. Which of the following statements is least likely to be true?

a) The man and his wife have three daughters
b) There were four sailors present on the preceding night
c) The passage is set in early September
d) People have lived in this area for millennia
e) The man has a heavy tool basket

4. Which of the following statements can be inferred to be true from the passage?

a) Someone has attempted to clear up the mess from the previous night
b) The man's wife threw her ring at him in a rage
c) Furmity is a classic dish of the region
d) The man likes to get drunk often
e) Several bottles of alcohol was opened the previous night

Verbal Reasoning Practice Question Answers

Passage 1: 3D Printing

1. **Can't Say:** The article describes some uses of 3D printing and also states that traditional injection moulding can be cheaper for producing high quantities of polymer products. It is impossible to tell with certainty whether 3D printers will take over from the older methods of manufacturing.

2. **True:** The final paragraph states that '3D printers give designers and concept development teams the ability to produce parts and concept models using a desktop size printer'. This is essentially saying that it is useful for producing prototype models and the statement is true.

3. **Can't Say:** 'Some techniques use two materials...'. The use of the word 'some' does not give us any indication of whether or not this is the most common technique.

4. **False:** The article states that 'The advantage of additive fabrication is its ability to produce **almost** any shape', implying that there are some that cannot be made.

Passage 2: A Damning Report for US Food Chains

1. **Can't Say:** The report concerns the calorific content of kids' menus throughout US restaurant-chains but **does not tell you anything about the general calorific consumption of US children.** This may or may not be true.

2. **Can't Say:** The statement from Hungry Joe's says that they 'offer a wide variety of kid's meals with healthier options and lower calories'. This may be true, but you can't tell how many customers choose them and how often they are served.

3. **Can't Say:** The information states that the milkshake at Ben's Bar and Grill is part of a combination meal that contains 1320 calories. It does not tell you which parts of the meal are high in calories. It may be that the milkshake is low in calories and the rest of the meal is responsible for the high calorie count - it's impossible to say.

4. **False:** According to the first paragraph, 430 calories is 1/3 of the recommended calorific intake for children aged 4-8.
430 x 3 is 1320 calories.

Passage 3: Big Brother is Watching You

1. **False:** The article does not indicate this. Firstly, in paragraph 2, the experiment is not about honesty, it is about generosity and the section tells us most people are not generous under anonymous circumstances. Secondly, paragraph 4 does describe an experiment assessing honesty but it only tells you that more people paid in the presence of a pair of eyes - nothing about whether they thought they were being watched and nothing about whether most people were dishonest without the eyes.

2. **False:** The game suggests this but... it's just a 'game' and not an 'experiment'. To state that evidence is reliable, it should not be an anecdote such as this. For experimental evidence to be deemed reliable it should generally come from a large randomised controlled trial - and certainly not a game!

3. **True:** The final paragraph suggests that we could use this effect to help reduce crime and anti-social behaviour.

4. **Can't Say**: In the article it states that 'It may be true that some images could reduce anti-social behaviour'. We therefore can't tell with any certainty, even though the rest of the article suggests that it probably is true.

Passage 4: Trial at The Hague

1. **Can't Say:** The judge says that Taylor is guilty of selling diamonds and buying weapons on behalf of the RUF. He has been found guilty of aiding and abetting war crimes for this. The passage gives no indication that Taylor ever entered Sierra Leone and we cannot say with certainty whether he committed atrocities there.

2. **True:** Jordi believes that part of the message that Taylor's jailing sends is that 'If you commit atrocities you will be held accountable.' It can be inferred that he believes Taylor committed atrocities.

3. **True:** This is clearly stated in the text.

4. **Can't Say:** Although the trial was hosted in Holland, it is impossible to tell whether judges of the Special Court for Sierra Leone were from Holland or not.

Passage 5: The Interpretation of Dreams

1. **True:** Jensen believes that 'it seems that conscience is silent in our dreams' and that we can commit crimes without remorse. Radestock is quoted as saying 'In dreams associations are effected without any influence of moral judgement'. The statement is true - both can be said to believe that moral judgement is suspended in dreams.

2. **Can't Say:** We are unable to tell what Freud believes from the passage. These are musings and he arrives at no personal conclusions.

3. **Can't Say:** Radestock notes that 'In dreams associations and ideas are combined without being effected by moral judgement'. There is no mention as to whether he has had dreams with immoral associations.

4. **Can't Say:** There is no mention of the frequency that dreams contain morally questionable behaviour. It may only be occasional, rather than 'usual'

Passage 6: Dutch Elm Disease

1. **Can't Say:** The article gives no information as to whether this is the case or not, although the survival of isolated pockets suggests it may be possible.

2. **True:** 20 million out of 30 million (2/3) of UK elms were dead 'within the decade' in an outbreak that started in the late 1960s.

3. **False:** In the 1950s, the first epidemic was over and the second had not yet started. As the first epidemic waned, Dr Peace had stated that 'unless the trend of the disease completely changes, the disaster that once seemed inevitable will not come to pass'.

4. **True:** Genes have been introduced from these trees to give European trees resistance. It follows that the Himalayan elms are resistant and not killed by the fungus.

Passage 7: Health Policy

1. **True:** Paterson is the health secretary and part of the government. In response to Paterson's proposals, the unions have called the government 'out of touch', implying that they think that Paterson is also out of touch.

2. **True:** The article states that there is 'only one group exempted: highly-paid managers'. Therefore doctors in richer parts of the country such as London would earn more than those working in less-well-off areas.

3. **Can't Say:** Even though this may be true, it is impossible to **tell from the passage** that this is the case. The criticism of Paterson by a liberal democrat spokesman would suggest the opposite if anything.

4. **False:** The Liberal Democrat spokesman says that this is 'a classic example of Paterson's ability to alienate the people he needs to rely on most - NHS staff' suggesting that this is not the first time he has been controversial with NHS staff

Passage 8: Never forget To Floss

1. **Can't Say:** The passage contains one anecdotal statement from Dr Kelly stating she 'often tells patients to include flossing as part of their routine'. However, there are two important points: firstly, she hints that people don't see it as important but doesn't emphatically state what percentage of her patients include it as part of their dental care routine. Moreover, one anecdotal report cannot be applied to the United States as a whole. If the statement read "Most patients in Dr Kelly's practice underestimate the importance of flossing as part of their dental care routine," the decision would be more difficult but the answer would still be "can't say" for the first reason.

2. **True:** The passage tells you that using matched pairs of twins helps to control for external variables.

3. **Can't tell:** 'Flossing in addition to brushing significantly lowers the levels of periodontal disease-causing bacteria compared with brushing alone.' We aren't told whether brushing alone reduces levels or not, so 'can't say' has to be the correct answer.

4. **False:** Treatment studies can be confounded by genetic factors. The fact that specific measures were taken to avoid this in the study suggest that this is more than a rare occurrence.

Passage 9: Snake Fangs

1. **Can't Say:** Vonk has looked at the embryology of fangs in snakes. We can't tell for certain whether he is a leading herpetologist from the passage (although this does seem likely). This would need to be explicitly stated for us to say it was true.

2. **True:** We are told that cobras and vipers have fangs at the front of their mouths. We are also told that they are the most venomous snakes. It is reasonable to deduce that frontal fangs are more venomous than fangs at the back.

3. **Can't Say:** We are told that 'Other types of snakes have fangs at the back of the mouth or even no fangs at all'. We aren't told that **all** other types of snakes have fangs at the back or not at all.

4. **True:** Both cobras and vipers 'use venom' (second paragraph) and it is safe to say that members of these families are venomous.

Passage 10: Twenty Thousand Leagues Under the Sea by Jules Verne, Chapter XIV

1. **Can't Say:** Conseil 'provides services' to the narrator, but we can't tell who, if anyone, employs him.

2. **True:** The 'ship's crew' are mentioned. We know that the Nautilus is under the surface between twenty five and thirty fathoms. We can therefore infer that the Nautilus is a 'ship under the sea' or a submarine.

3.**True:** He is giving the 'perfect liberty' and ensuring they are delicately and abundantly fed. As the Captain of the ship, we can assume he has ultimate control of how his guests are being looked after.

4. **Can't Say:** This may be true, but he may have decided that he does not wish to see them at present.

Passage 11: The Adventure of the Copper Beeches by Sir Arthur Conan Doyle

Top tip: It can be difficult to think exactly what 'least likely to be true' means. You can also think of it as 'most likely to be false'.

1. **e)** Miss Hunter came to see Sherlock Holmes because she had no relations to turn to for advice. It is highly likely that she considers him to be trustworthy. We can't tell whether Miss Stoper owns the Westaway business and although it seems likely that Miss Hunter wanted to go to Halifax with the Colonel, there is no indication given in the script that this may be the case. The stout mans says 'That one may do' indicating he is not sure that she is exactly what he is looking for. Miss Hunter is looking for work from Miss Stoper and is not going to be working for her.

2. **c)** The fact that there are enough unemployed governesses to keep an agency busy looking for work for them suggests that many women wished to work as governesses at that time. None of the other statements can be inferred definitively from the passage.

3. **e)** Miss Hunter talks of the Colonel's children, implying more than one, so this statement must be false. We can't tell if Colonel Munro is American or not, whether the stout man has bad intentions towards Miss Hunter or if Sherlock Holmes is tired. Sherlock Holmes states that he would be happy to do anything to serve Miss Hunter, so we can assume that he wishes to help her.

4. **b)** Miss Hunter was employed by the Colonel for five years and only left his service because he moved away, suggesting that she was an effective governess. The obese man is at an agency that hires governesses who are mostly young women. Miss Hunter has no close relations and has the look of someone that has had to 'make their own way in life' so probably did not have an easy start to life. Sherlock Holmes is willing to listen and help Miss Hunter so he most likely likes her. Miss Hunter is neatly dressed and so probably takes care over her appearance.

Passage 12: The War On Smoking

1. **True:** The passage tells you that the epidemic has developed faster than any previous forecasts. Therefore, the rate of smoking uptake must be greater than previously predicted. By deduction the previous forecast must have been wrong.

2. **Can't Say:** The passage states that chronic obstructive pulmonary disease is a more common cause of smoking-related deaths in China than in the West, but does not tell you the differences between the most common causes of smoking or non-smoking related illnesses between the two regions.

3. **Can't Say:** Smoking increases the risk of lung cancer and our own knowledge may tell us that the statement is true.. However, the question relates to what can be deduced from the passage. We are not told the proportion of cases of lung cancer that are related to smoking and therefore are unable to tell whether 'lung cancer is **usually** caused by smoking'.

4. **True:** The war on smoking is 'being won' in the West. The next statement relates this sentence to the worldwide death toll increasing overall 'as poorer countries step in'. It is therefore reasonable to conclude that if the war is 'being won', this means the death toll is reducing in the West. 'Developing' or poorer countries are 'stepping in' and keeping the death toll increasing, so the statement is true.

Passage 13: Transistor Radios

1. **Can't Say:** Transistor radios became the most popular **electronic** communication device in history. Although our knowledge may tell us that this means they may well be the most popular communication device in history, we cannot tell this from the passage. It could be argued that the voice is the most popular communication device in history!

2. **False:** 'Virtually all commercial broadcast receivers are now transistor based'. 'Transistors are current amplifiers, rather than voltage amplifiers'.

3. **Can't Say:** Post-war prosperity was one of the factors associated with the increased the popularity of transistor radios. From the passage, it cannot be said to be the biggest cause.

4. **Can't Say:** Boom boxes are given as an example of 'other portable media players' which 'took over' from transistor radios in the 1970s. It is not possible to tell whether boom boxes were more popular than transistor radios. It may have been that the numbers of boom boxes and cassette players combined was larger than transistor radios.

Passage 14: A Mayor's Vision

1. **True:** The second paragraph explains that sentiments derived from poor housing and amenities have recently led to acts of terrorism.

2. **Can't Say:** The text states that he is 'only 36 years old' but not that he was the youngest ever mayor of Karachi

3. **True:** This is a reasonable conclusion to derive given that he has gone out of his way to ease congestion and that he wants his city to 'become 'world class': "In order to ease congestion he has completed six under and over-passes together with a signal-free crosstown corridor."

4. **True:** This is a reasonable conclusion to draw. Although the second paragraph cites only an opinion that many believe him to be out of touch, there is substantial evidence later in the text to support this: suicide bombings, terrorist acts and a lack of control supported by evidence given in the final paragraph concerning the administrative structures in place.

Passage 15: Alcohol-Related Illness

1. **True:** 811,443 / 1.71 = 474,528

2. **Can't Say:** The passage tells you that the definition is wider and encompasses a greater number of conditions than that previously used in other reports. Whilst this is a likely contributing factor to the increase in observed frequency of related diseases you cannot be certain this is the case. This is because you do not know which definitions have been excluded or included or the frequency of diseases within those categories. For example, if the criteria were redefined to include two extra categories and exclude another, you might expect the observed frequency to increase. However, the sum of the frequencies within the two may be less than the total within the excluded category. Paradoxically, therefore, using the same definition across study years may even result in an increase in the observed difference.

3. **Can't Say:** Although we are told that alcoholic liver disease is at an all time high in England, we aren't told how it is in the rest of the UK. It may be higher in Scotland, Wales or Northern Ireland.

4. **False:** The information that we are given in the passage is that 'similar strategies in the US have failed to produce significant results'. The evidence we have that this is not 'likely'. Had the question been 'Forcing manufacturers to put warnings on will reduce alcoholic liver disease' the answer would have been 'can't tell'.

Passage 16: Black Holes

1. **True:** This is clearly stated in the first sentence: 'A black hole is a region of space-time from which nothing can escape'.
Often, statements which use words like 'impossible' are not true as there are often exceptions. It takes an absolute statement such as the one given to be able to draw this conclusion with certainty.

2. True: The theory of general relativity predicts the existence of black holes. An event horizon is an effect of a black hole. General relativity therefore has to be used to predict the existence of an 'event horizon', which would not exist without a black hole.

3. **Can't Say:** Although black holes are 'expected' to form when very massive stars collapse, there is no indication whether this is a rare of common event

4. True: 'Nothing can escape from gravity'. This includes light and 'blue light'.

Passage 17: Glacier Retreat

1. **True:** The team sent field-workers to measure glaciers manually to ensure their data was accurate. These can be considered to be 'careful measures.'

2. Can't Say: The article gives data for what has happened over the last 40 years. There is no information regarding what was happening before this

3. True: The passage states that glaciers in the south have a higher rate of retreat. It also states that the Ecrins massif is to the south of the Mont Blanc massif and so it can be deduced that glaciers in the Ecrins are retreating quicker than in the Mont Blanc massif.

4. Can't Say: Although this seems likely, there is no specific information in the passage to expand from the Alps to the rest of the world. In reality, this is true (with a few notable exceptions).

Passage 18: Hardangervidda

1. Can't Say: Given the cold climate it is likely that cross-country skiing takes place in other seasons such as the Spring, but we can't say for certain from the information given in the article.

2. True: The Hardangervidda national park is 'entirely above 1000m'. This suggests it consists of only the plateau. The national park extends in to the county of Hordaland and therefore some of the plateau (as implied in the first paragraph) is found within Hordaland.

3. True: The National Park is found entirely above 1000m. The landscape is 'treeless' on the plateau. Therefore the tree line must be below 1000m.

4. Can't Say: This information is not given in the text, but it may be true. We 'can't say'.

Passage 19: It's Still Wine

1. True: You are told in the second paragraph that the weight of the receptacle has a significant impact on the amount of energy required for transportation, and therefore the cost. You are also told in the final paragraph that a plastic pouch only weighs one twentieth of its glass counterpart, set against one eight for a plastic bottle. The costs involved would therefore be substantially less.

2. Can't Say: The passage tells you that papsaks are out of favour in South Africa due to a specific reason concerning social disruption. It doesn't tell you how things would be different in England

3. Can't Say: The reason given that plastic pouches are better for the environment is that they are lighter and therefore require less energy to transport. No information is given on the energy used in production of either.

4. Can't Say: Although 'many wine connoisseurs throw their arms up in abhorrence at the very notion of drinking wine from a plastic bottle' we are not told why. It may be simply they prefer the feel of a glass bottle.

Passage 20: Neurobiology – Hearing Movement!

1. True This can be reasonably inferred from the passage. Since you are told that this arises as a result of cross-activated senses and are given similar examples, this would be a logical deduction.

2. Can't Say Only individuals with auditory synesthesia outperformed normal individuals in this particular type of test in the study; we don't know what the data is for visual synaesthetes.

3. True The study quoted was small, involving only 4 synaesthetes, so it is almost certainly not statistically significant. However, it points to the conclusion that they probably are better, so from the information given this statement can be said to be true.

4. Can't Say Although the article is about auditory synesthesia, it does mention other types. There is no indication how common these are relative to each other. The article also states 'very little is known about the phenomenon of synesthesia'.

Passage 21: 20 000 Leagues Under the Sea, by Jules Verne, Chapter XXX

1. d) 'The Nautilus made two brief stops on its passage through the Mediterranean' is most likely to be false. We are told that the Captain only brought the vessel to the surface at night to renew the air and was keen to be out of the Mediterranean. Although we cannot tell for certain whether the other statements are true or false, they are more likely to be true than false.

2. b) It is clearly stated that the Mediterranean is 'distasteful' to the Captain. It is possible that Ned Land is trying to escape and that Michelet was a famous French travel writer, however these are not apparent from the text. It is apparent that the Nautilus is travelling very fast and this is the statement ' The Captain is pushing the Nautilus to it's top speed' is most likely to be true.

3. b) The distance travelled is six hundred leagues – the 'estimated course' which took forty-eight hours. This is the distance from Greece to the Straits of Gibraltar and it is not possible that the Nautilus would travel at a depth of even a sixth of this distance. The other statements are either true or we are unable to tell for certain that they are false.

4. **e)** The Nautilus only needs to surface at night. Even though it is winter, there will be at least 8 hours of light in the Mediterranean and this statement must be true. We cannot tell for certain whether the other statements are true or false.

Passage 22 Chapter 2, The Mayor of Casterbridge by Thomas Hardy

1. b) The passage states that the man arrived with his family and that 'little' Elizabeth-Jane has gone with his wife and the sailor. This implies that she is likely to be his daughter. The man can remember some of the previous night and it seems unlikely that he was happily married if he sold his wife. We don't know whether furmity is usually mixed with rum or not and there is no indication how likely the man is to find his wife again.

2. d) The only one of these statements that can be said to be definitely false, as the man wakes up in a marquee, not a shed.

3. a) The passage refers to the man's 'family' and only one daughter is mentioned. Had there been other daughters, he would have probably referred to them as well. This makes this statement marginally less likely than the fact there were four sailors present the preceding night – we have no indication of the numbers. The passage could easily be set in early September and prehistoric forts are referred to, indicating that people have lived in the area for 'millennia'. The man has to 'shoulder the tool basket' and it is probably heavy.

4. e) 'Corks dot the grassy floor' and the man is awaking from a drunken stupor – this implies that several bottles of alcohol were opened the previous night. There is no evidence that the man likes to get drunk often, that furmity is a dish of the region or how the ring ended up on the floor. It seems unlikely, given the mess described, that someone has tried to clear up.

Chapter 2

Quantitative Reasoning

Quantitative Reasoning

What is it?

UKCAT says: This subtest 'assesses your ability to use numerical skills to solve problems. It assumes familiarity with the numbers to the standard of a good pass at GCSE. However, items are less to do with numerical facility and more to do with problem solving'.

You are given 25 minutes to read the instructions (1 minute allowed) and answer 36 items associated with data in the form of tables, charts and/or graphs. This means you have approximately 40 seconds per question.

This part of the test looks at your ability to analyse data and solve simple numerical problems. The sort of things you could be asked to do include:

- Addition, subtraction, multiplication and division.
- Calculation of percentages.
- Analysis of data in the form of graphs and tables
- Simple calculations involving speed, distance, time and areas

Certain topics are favourites of the examiners. Questions often relate to money, currencies and taxes, travelling times, fuel consumption and business costs.

Questions are formatted in one of several different ways. We have provided worked examples of each style.

- Plain text containing numerical data
- Graphs and/or tables containing numerical data. Very often there is text accompanying the data containing further information relevant to the question.

Why is Quantitative reasoning included in the UKCAT?

Professional life often involves processing large amounts of data; very often this data is numerical. Basic skills are required such as doing simple sums and interpreting graphs, for example when prescribing for children, you often need to calculate the dose of a medicine per kg of the child's weight. Tables of data very often appear in journals. Audits require basic manipulation of data. The ability to critically interpret and manipulate data is essential for your future professional career.

Top Tips:

- *Read the scenario and look at the data to get an overall view of what the data is about*
- *Check **ALL** of the **units** - these may need converting. Use the figures give rather than any you may already know.*
- *Know how to use the on-screen calculator and the note board and pen provided. You can practice using the calculator online.*
- *Make sure you are happy with percentages, averages, fractions and ratios*
- *Eliminate obviously wrong answers if you are struggling and then choose the most likely remaining answer*
- *Make sure you **stick to time**. It is always worth 'flagging' the ones you are unsure of to come back to, but if you do this make sure you have at least ticked one of the answers before your time runs out. Remember there is no negative marking so never leave a blank answer!*
- ***Practice as many questions as you can under timed conditions.***

Worked Examples:

Example 1

Mr X cycled from his house to Brighton in 2 hours 15 minutes. He had three 5 minute rests. When he left, the reading on his odometer was 1086 miles. When he arrived the reading on his odometer was 1108 miles.

1. What was Mr X's average speed whilst cycling?

5.5 mph
8.8 mph
9.8 mph
11 mph~
22 mph

Answer: 11 mph

Speed = Distance / Time
1108 - 1086 = 22 miles
Total rest time = 5 minutes x 3 = 15 minutes
Total cycling time = 2 hours 15 minutes - 15 minutes = 2 hours

Average speed = 22/2 = 11 miles per hour

2. One kilometre (km) is equivalent to 0.6214 miles. How many kilometres has Mr X's bike done when he arrives in Brighton?

35.4 km
688.5 km
1747.7 km
1772.8 km
1783.1 km

Answer: 1783.1 km

1108 / 0.6214 = 1783.1 km

3. Mr X can do the same journey in 38 minutes by car. How much faster is Mr X's average driving speed compared to his average cycling speed?

17.9 mph
22.1 mph
23.7 mph
24.9 mph
38.2 mph

Answer: 23.7mph faster

22 miles / 38 minutes = 0.579 miles / minute
0.579 x 60 = 34.7 mph average driving speed
34.7 - 11 = 23.7 mph faster

4. Mr X bought the bike when it had 483 miles on the odometer. Mr Y has borrowed Mr X's bike twice to cycle to and from work. Mr Y lives 6 miles from work. Mr X has never leant the bike to anyone else. What is the total number of miles Mr X has ridden on his bike since owning it when he arrives in Brighton?

579 miles
601 miles
613 miles
619 miles
625 miles

Answer: 601 miles

Number of miles on the bike when arrived in Brighton = 1108
Total number of miles Mr X has ridden on the bike = 1108 - 483 - (6 x 2 x 2) = 601 miles

The main difficulty here is reading the question carefully enough to make sure you do the right calculation. This is the last question of four, so if you find yourself spending too much time on it, guess an answer and flag it and come back later if you have time. As you can see the difficulties here lie not in the sums themselves, but in identifying the correct data to use to answer the question quickly. The questions often tend to get progressively harder through the scenario.

Example 2:

A company is employed to collect blood samples from local GP surgeries and deliver them to the hospital laboratory. The table below shows the number of surgeries at certain distances from the hospital. Each GP surgery serves on average 12,000 patients.

Distance From Hospital (km)	Number of GP Surgeries
<5	15
5-9	5
10-14	23
15-19	11
>20	8

1. How many surgeries does the company collect samples from?

15
54
62
68
71

Answer: 62

This requires you to simply extract the data from the table:
15+5+23+11+8 = 62

2. Estimate how many people are registered with a GP within 5km of the hospital.

120,000
180,000
205,000
744,000
Can't tell

Answer: 180,000

There are 15 surgeries within 5 km of the hospital and we are told that each surgery has an average of 12,000 registered patients.
So, 15 x 12,000 = 180,000

3. Calculate the total population within 25km.

498,000
500,000
620,000
744,000
Can't say

Answer: Can't say

We can't tell how many of the 8 surgeries that are more than 20km away are within 25km of the hospital, so although 62 x 12,000 = 744,000 we can't say this with certainty so should answer 'Can't say'.

4. 12 km away is a city of 120,000 people. What is the approximate population (registered with a GP) that lives 10-14km away from the hospital but not in the city?

0
83,000
156,000
264,000
276,000

Answer: 156,000

Total population that lives within 10-14km away = 23 x 12,000 = 276,000
276,000 - 120,000 = 156,000

As you can see, the calculations themselves do not require great knowledge of mathematics! The difficulty is in answering them accurately in the time allowed.

Quantitative Reasoning Exercise

Try and do the following questions under 'timed conditions'. Allow yourself 1 minute for the instructions and then 12 minutes to answer the 20 questions that follow. Answers are at the end of the section. As a rough guide, take 10 - 20 seconds to scan the data and then 30-40 seconds to answer each question, checking back to the appropriate part of the text as required. The instructions are similar to those you will encounter in the real test.

An explanation is provided with the answer to each question.

Take 1 minute to read these instructions.

You will be presented with data at the top of the question. For each data set, there will be four questions, each with five possible answers.

Answer 20 questions in 12 minutes. Try and answer all the questions as there is no negative marking.

Llaned District General Hospital

A hospital manager is looking at the costs of running wards in the first and second quarters of the year and draws up the following table.

Ward	Expected Average Running Cost/Week	Actual Cost per 1st Quarter (Jan-Mar)	Actual Cost per 2nd Quarter (Apr-Jun)
A	12,000	156,000	189,000
B	40,000	300,000	336,000
C	9,000	96,000	90,000
D	16,000	213,000	204,000
E	33,000	426,000	420,000
F	18,000	63,000	62,000

All costs are in pounds.
Assume January to June inclusive is 26 weeks and each quarter is 13 weeks.

1. By how much have the running costs for Ward D exceeded those for Ward C in the first six months of this year?

£168,000
£182,000
£216,000
£231,000
None of the above

2. How much is ward A over budget in the first 6 months of the year?

£0
£33,000
£120,000
£189,000
£333,000

3. What was the difference between the actual cost and the expected cost per week in the 2nd quarter for ward E?

£231
£692
£923
£6000
£32,308

4. Ward D gets a new manager who thinks that she can reduce the costs of the ward's 2nd quarter by 15%. What is her expected average running cost per week for the 3rd quarter?

£12,089
£13,338
£13,645
£13,600
£14,981

Buying shares: Lucky Mining Company

Time Period	Total Profit (%)
1 day	0.05
1 week	-1.18
1 month	10.03
3 months	36.27
6 months	42.96
1 year	64.88
3 years	111.33
5 years	112.98
10 years	107.92

The table shows the percentage of profit an investor would have made depending on when they had invested their money in the Lucky Mining Company. For example, had an investor bought shares 3 months ago, they would have made a profit of 36.27%. Had they bought shares 3 years ago, they would have made a profit of 111.33%.

1. Mr J bought 200 shares 6 months ago for £680. What are his shares worth now?

£4.86
£292.13
£926.64
£972.13
£1121.18

2. What was the value of one of Mr J's shares 1 year ago?

180p
281p
295p
412p
486p

3. Mr R bought £800 of shares 10 years ago. What were his shares worth 5 years ago?

£701.11
£764.17
£780.99
£785.91
£837.51

66

4. What would £10,000 of shares bought 10 years ago have been worth one week ago?

£11020
£20674
£20792
£20910
£21040

Buying a Car

Richard has narrowed his choice of second-hand cars down to 5 models, shown in the table.

He plans to drive 10,000 miles per year and expects to own the car for 30 months. He drives the same number of miles each month,

The dealer says that if he sells the car, he will be able to get 50% of what he initially paid after 30 months.

None of the cars are currently taxed. Tax is a one-off annual charge and varies from model to model (shown in the table).

Car Type	Price	Tax/year	Miles per gallon
Matrix	7,000	80	60
Zephyr	6,495	100	45
Chilli	8,000	80	58
Mayo	7,450	140	38
Lexacor	6,995	145	36

Fuel costs 141.9p per litre and does not change. One gallon is 4.55 litres.
All prices in the table are in pounds.

1. How much would he expect to spend on fuel over the first two years if he bought a Zephyr?

£630.66
£1434.75
£2438.76
£2869.50
£2912.18

2. Which car represents the least cost for Richard over the period he owns it?

Matrix
Zefyr
Chilli
Mayo
Lexacor

3. Richard decides to buy a Chilli. If he does manage to sell it for the expected price after 30 months, what will his total expenditure have been?

£4851.63
£6982.92
£7022.92
£8851.63
£11,022.92

4. By adding 'Superfuel' mix he can improve the mileage per gallon of the Chilli by 10%. Superfuel mix costs £4.50 and he needs to add it every 1000 miles. How much would it save him for his first 1000 miles?

£0.40
£1.15
£5.65
£9.48
£10.15

Sailing Boat

Colin owns a sailing boat. He decides to sail from Holetown to Point Lebacca. One knot is equal to one nautical mile per hour. One nautical mile is equal to 1852m. Assume that he sails in a straight line from point to point and is unaffected by tides.

1. He sets sail at 1000 hrs from Holetown and sails across the bay directly towards Point Lebacca, initially at a speed of 6 knots. He covers a distance of 3 nautical miles. The wind then picks up and he travels 5 nautical miles at a speed of 10 knots and arrives at Point Lebacca. At what time did he arrive?

1100 hrs
1200 hrs
1230 hrs
1300 hrs
1330 hrs

2. When he arrives at Point Lebacca he drops anchor and has lunch for one and a half hours. The wind picks up even more and he is able to sail straight back to Holetown at an average speed of 12 knots. At what time does he arrive back?

1140 hrs
1240 hrs
1310 hrs
1340 hrs
1410 hrs

3. How many kilometres is it to sail directly from Holetown to Point Lebacca and back?

8.0 km
14.816 km
18.520km
29.632 km
35.882 km

4. By using the motor Colin can add an extra 6.4 knots to his average speed. Had he used his motor on this trip, how long would the journey there and back have taken him?

48 minutes
1 hour
1 hour and 8 minutes
1 hour 23 minutes
2 hours and 40 minutes

Growing Vegetables

A farmer decides to plot how many kilograms of different types of vegetables he grows for two consecutive years. Look at the chart below and answer the following questions:

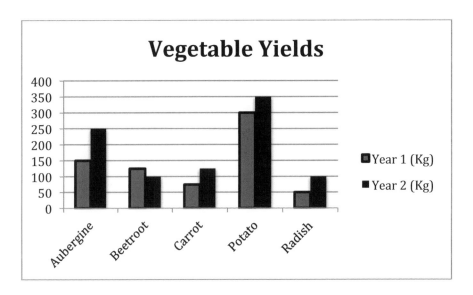

1. Which vegetable saw the biggest percentage increase in yield between years 1 and 2?

Aubergine
Beetroot
Carrot
Potato
Radish

2. The beetroot crop was affected by a disease known as beetroot blight in year 2. Around the country, average yields fell by 25% from the year 1. By what percentage did beetroot yields fall at this farm?

15%
20%
25%
30%
50%

3. The chart below shows the price of each type of vegetable in year 2.

Vegetable	Price / Kg (£)	Production cost /Kg (£)
Aubergine	2.20	1.00
Beetroot	0.50	0.10
Carrot	0.25	0.10
Potato	0.10	0.09
Radish	1.10	0.70

80% of the aubergines produced were sold. How much profit did the farmer make from aubergines in year 2?

£144
£240
£300
£350
£1200

4. Which of the vegetables cost the most to produce in year 2?

Aubergine
Beetroot
Carrot
Potato
Radish

Answers:

Llaned District General Hospital

1. £231,000

Total cost for ward D = £213,000 + £204,000 = £417,000
Total cost for ward C = £96,000 + £90,000 = £186,000
The difference in cost is therefore £471,000 - £186,000 = £231,000

2. £33,000:

Actual cost = £156,000 + £189,000 = £345,000
Expected cost = 12,000 x 26 = £312,000
£345,000-£312,000 = £33,000

3. £692

Expected cost : 33,000
Actual cost: 420,000 / 13 = 32307.7 = £32,308
£33,000 - £32308 = £692 less per week

4. £13,338

In the 2nd quarter, ward D cost £204,000.
The total cost in the next quarter is £204,000 x 0.85 = £173,400
£173,400 / 13 = expected cost per week = £13338

Buying shares: Lucky Mining Company

1. £972.13

£680 x 1.4296 = £972.13

2. 295p

Current value of 200 shares = £972.13
Current value of 1 share = £972.13 / 200 = £4.86
Shares have risen 64.88% since one year ago, so £4.86/1.6488 = £2.95 = 295p

3. £780.99

Over the last 10 years, the shares have increased in value by 107.92 %.
The increase from 5 years ago is 112.98%, implying the value of the shares
went down between 10 and 5 years ago.

Current value = £800 x 2.0792 = £1663.36
Value 5 years ago = £1663.36 / 2.1298 = £780.99

If you were running out of time at this point, it is easy to eliminate anything
above £800, as you can tell from the table the shares must have gone down in
value to be able to make more of a profit had you invested 5 years ago
compared to 10 years ago. The extra profit is not great, so you can easily
eliminate £701.11, leaving you only 3 possible answers to choose from.

4. £21040

Current value of the shares: £10,000 x 2.0792 = £20792
Had shares been bought 1 week ago, there would have been a drop in value of
1.18%, i.e. shares are worth 98.82% of what they were worth last week. so
£20792 / 0.9882 = £21040

Buying a Car

1. £2869.50

10,000 miles/yr x 2 = 20,000 miles total.
20,000 miles at 45 miles per gallon = 20,000/45 = number of gallons = 444.44
gallons
4.55 x 444.44 = 2022.2 litres
Cost per litre = 141.9p
2022.2 x 141.9 = 286950p = £2869.50

2. Matrix

There is no need to do any calculations. From the table, the Matrix has the best
miles per gallon and the lowest tax. The only one that could possibly be better
value is the Zephyr. However, we know that it does 25% fewer miles per gallon.
Given that we expect Richard to spend £2869.50 on fuel over two years if he
were to use the Zephyr, the saving in expenditure on fuel will more than cover
the difference in expenditure on price.

3. £7022.92

Initial price = £8,000
Tax = £80 x 3 years = £240
Fuel = 25,000 miles / 58 = 431.03 gallons
431.03 x 4.55 = 1961.19 litres =
1961.19 x 141.9 = 278292p = £2782.92p

Sells the car for £8000 x 0.50 = £4,000

Total expenditure = 8000 + 240 + 2782.92 - 4000 = £7022.92

4. £5.65
Total cost without Superfuel for 1000 miles = 1000 / 58 = 17.24 gallons
17.24 x 4.55 = 78.45 litres
78.45 x 141.9p = 11132p

Total cost with Superfuel for 1000 miles = 1000 / (58 + 5.8) = 15.67 gallons
15.67 x 4.55 = 71.30 litres
71.30 x 141.9 = 10117p + cost of super fuel (450p) = 10567p

11132 - 10567 = 565p = £5.65 saving for one thousand miles

Sailing Boat

1. 1100 hrs

Speed = Distance / Time and so Time = Distance / Speed

In this case:
3 nautical miles / 6 knots = 1/2 hr
5 nautical miles / 10 knots = 1/2 hr
Therefore if he sets off at 1000 hrs, he arrives at 1100 hrs.

2. 1310 hrs

Time to sail back = 8 nautical miles / 12 knots = 2/3 hour = 40 minutes
He arrived at 1100 hrs and departed one and a half hours later at 1230 hrs.
He therefore arrived back at Holetown at 1310 hrs.

3. 29.632km

Total distance is (5 + 3 nautical miles) x 2 (return journey)
16 x 1852m = 29,632m = 29.632 km

4. 1 hour

Average speed without motor = 16 nautical miles in 1 hr 40 minutes = 16 /
1.6666 = 9.6 knots
Average speed with motor = 9.6 knots + 6.4 knots = 16 knots

Time = distance / speed = 16 nautical miles / 16 knots = 1 hour

Growing Vegetables

1. Radishes

Radishes mass was doubled in year 2, a 100% increase.

2. 20%

Beetroot yield in year 1 was 125kg and in year 2 100kg.
The fall was therefore 25kg.
25kg / 125kg x 100% = 20%

3. £240

250kg of aubergines produced and 80% sold = 200kg produced.
200kg sold at a profit of £1.20 (£2.20 - £1)
200 x 1.2 = £240

4. Aubergines

You do not have to do any calculations to work this out quickly. The most
expensive to produce per kg are aubergines. Potatoes were the only vegetable
that were produced in more quantity, but cost less than a tenth per kilogram to
produce compared to aubergines.

Quantitative Reasoning Practice Questions

Allow 2 minutes and 40 seconds for each set of 4 questions.
For 2 sets, allow 5 minutes and 20 seconds.
For 5 sets, allow 13 minutes and 20 seconds.
For 9 sets, allow 24 minutes.

1. Travelling to Chamonix

You wish to travel from your home in Gloucester, UK to Chamonix, France for a week's skiing. There are two airports nearby, Bristol and Cardiff, both offering flights to Geneva, Switzerland from where it is a short bus or train ride to Chamonix. Below are some details for the journey:

	Distance	Cost	Time
Gloucester – Cardiff (car)	74.6 miles	£8.95 (fuel only)	1 hr 38 mins
Gloucester – Bristol (car)	46.7 miles	£5.60 (fuel only)	1 hr 00 mins
Bristol – Geneva (plane)	730.9 miles	£95.80	1 hr 12 mins
Cardiff – Geneva (plane)	763.8 miles	£65	1 hr 15 mins
Geneva – Chamonix (bus)	81.7 km	20 Euro	0 hr 58 mins
Geneva – Chamonix (train)	81.7 km	15 Euro	0 hr 49 mins

1. You have been advised to arrive at Cardiff airport 90 minutes before the flight takes off and expect to wait 30 minutes for a bus or train from Geneva to Chamonix. What is the shortest possible time for the journey when travelling via Cardiff?

a) 181 minutes
b) 3 hrs 42 minutes
c) 4 hrs 08 minutes
d) 346 minutes
e) 5 hrs 42 minutes

76

2. The Geneva to Chamonix bus does 20km for one gallon of fuel. How many more miles per gallon does the car do compared to the bus? (One gallon costs £6.26; One mile is 1609 metres)

a) 0 miles
b) 3 miles
c) 39.8 miles
d) 74.6 miles
e) 94.2 miles

3. The current exchange rate is 1.2 Euros per Pound. What is the cheapest possible total fare to Chamonix?

a) £118.07
b) £88.95
c) £73.95
d) £86.45
e) 142 Euros

4. What is the shortest distance it is possible to travel? (There are 1609 metres in a mile)

a) 3085 km
b) 828.38 miles
c) 1,430,690 metres
d) 889.18 miles
e) 1430 km

2. Cycling Speed

A cyclist sets out to ride between points 'A' and 'B'. The speed she travels at each point of her journey are drawn on the chart below and she reaches point B in 5 hours.

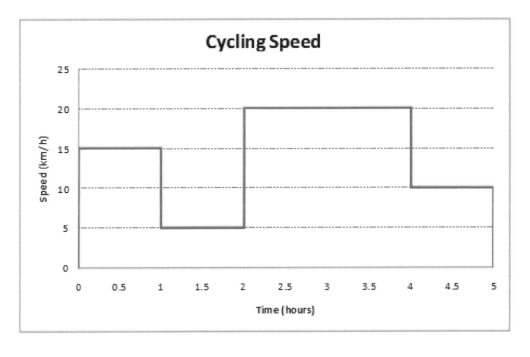

1. How far is she from point A at 3.5 hours into her journey?

a) 5.7km
b) 13km
c) 20km
d) 33km
e) 50km

During leg 1 she travels 15 x 1 = 15 km
During leg 2 she travels 5 x 1 = 5 km
During leg 3 she travels 20 x 1.5 = 30 km
Total distance = 50km

2. What is the distance between point A and point B?

a) 33.3km
b) 45km
c) 50km
d) 60km
e) 70km correct

3. Assuming she always travels at a constant speed, how much faster must she travel between 1 and 2 hours into her journey in order to reach point B in only 4.5 hours as opposed to 5?

a) 0km/h
b) 5km/h
c) 10km/h
d) 15km/h
e) None of the above

4. Another cyclist completes the same journey, but travels 20 km/h whilst our first cyclist is travelling at 15km/h and 15km/h whilst our first cyclist is travelling 10km/h. How long does it take the second cyclist to complete the same journey?

a) 3 hours and 55 minutes
b) 4 hours
c) 4 hours and 25 minutes
d) 4 hours and 30 minutes
e) Can't say

3. Dunvoor Ferry Timetable

Monday to Saturday

Depart East Valbride	Depart Logan Point
0630	0640
0650	0700
20 min intervals	20 min intervals
0850	0840
0915	0900
30 min intervals	0930
2045	30 min intervals
2110	2100
2130	2120

Sunday

0845	0830
30 min intervals	30 min intervals
2045	2100
2110	2120
2130	-------

Crossing times are 95 minutes. The return journey is 120 miles. All ferries are required to wait 1 hour and 15 minutes at either port for unloading, refuelling and reloading.

1. Assume a constant speed. At what speed does the ferry travel?

a) 19 miles per hour
b) 26 miles per hour
c) 38 miles per hour
d) 63 miles per hour
e) 76 miles per hour

2. A ferry leaves East Valbride for the first run on Sunday morning. At what time would it depart Logan point for the return journey?

a) 1030
b) 1100
c) 1130
d) 1200
e) 1230

3. The ferry captain wants to sail his ferry to Logan point and return at 09:00 to East Valbride. What time must he leave East Valbride?

a) 0630
b) 0650
c) 0720
d) 0850
e) None of the above

4. Ben has an interview at 10.20 AM on a Tuesday in East Valbride. He lives in Logan point and wishes to arrive at least 30 minutes early. Which ferry is the latest he should catch?

a) 0740
b) 0750
c) 0800
d) 0815
e) 0820

4. Fence Painting

Mrs Gleason needs to repaint her fence. She has found a colour of paint that she likes but the cost of this is much higher than an ordinary white-wash so she has decided to start with a short section of fence - the dimensions and size of which is given below. The decorating panels along the top of the fence are perfect semicircles with a radius of 0.3m.

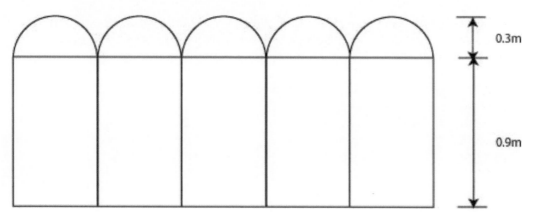

Use Pi to 5 decimal figures: 3.14159

1. What is the total area of **semi-circular fence decoration only** that Mrs Gleason needs to paint?

a) 0.71 m²
b) 0.94 m²
c) 1.41. m²
d) 1.88 m²
e) 9.42 m²

2. What is the total area of the main fence panelling **(not including the semi-circular decorative panelling)** that Mrs Gleason needs to paint?

a) 0.27 m²
b) 0.54 m²
c) 1.35 m²
d) 2.70 m²
e) 3.41 m²

3. What is the total area of **the entire fence** that Mrs Gleason needs to paint?

a) 3.41 m^2
b) 3.64 m^2
c) 4.11 m^2
d) 4.58 m^2
e) 12.12 m^2

4. Mrs Gleason particularly likes Modson's purple hue and wishes to paint her fence in this colour The paint only comes in 1.5 litre pots and 1 litre covers approximately 10m^2. How much paint is she going to have left over?

a) 0.10L
b) 0.34L
c) 0.78L
d) 0.99L
e) 1.30L

5. Flying

Below is the timetable for two different airlines who operate routes from London to Delhi. All times are local.

Air Austria (daily flights except Tuesdays)

London - Vienna	Vienna - Delhi	Price
Depart 0915 Arrive 1240	Depart 1315 Arrive 0005	£521.50

Air Abu Dhabi (daily flights)

London – Abu-Dhabi	Abu-Dhabi – Delhi	Price
Depart 0915 Arrive 1920	Depart 2230 Arrive 0330	£543.37

At midnight in London it is 0100 in Vienna, 0400 in Abu Dhabi and 0530 in Delhi.

Both airlines fly at an average speed of 600mph.

1. How much longer does it take to go to Delhi via Abu Dhabi compared to going via Vienna?

82

a) No extra time
b) 1 hr 55 mins
c) 3 hrs 25 mins
d) 3 hrs 35 mins
e) 5 hrs 30 mins

2. Both airlines fly at an average speed of 600mph. What is the distance from London to Vienna?

a) 900 miles
b) 1450 miles
c) 1550 miles
d) 2305 miles
e) 30,000 miles

3. What is the total flying time from London to Delhi via Abu Dhabi?

a) 8 hrs 10 mins
b) 9hrs 15 mins
c) 9 hrs 35 mins
d) 12 hrs 45 mins
e) 18 hrs 15 mins

4. What is the cost per mile when flying from London to Delhi via Abu Dhabi?

a) 94p/mile
b) 91p/mile
c) 9.1p/mile
d) 9.4p/mile
e) £1.63/mile

6. Moon Limited

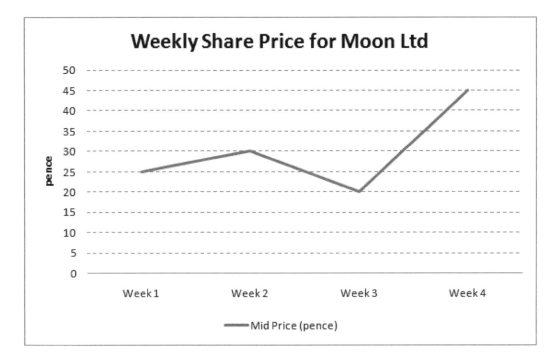

The mid price is calculated as halfway between the open price on the stock market at 8 am on Monday morning and the close price for the week at 5pm on Friday.

1. A financial analyst wishes to know the return on his investment. It is then end of week 4, assuming he bought and sold at the mid-price, what profit did he make (in £) if he bought 100 shares in week 2?

a) £4.28
b) £8.57
c) £15.00
d) £20.03
e) None of the above

2. An investor with £12000 to invest buys shares in week 2 when the price is 30 pence per share. If the share price increases by 50% every 2 weeks, how much will his investment be worth in 6 weeks?

84

a) £18,000
b) £40,500
c) £54,000
d) £72,000
e) £150,000

3. An investor invests £5000 at week 1. He takes out half of what is left in week 3 and puts it in a savings account. He then takes the rest out in week 4 and puts that in his savings account too. What is his total profit? (All transactions were at the mid-price)

a) £600
b) £1500
c) £2400
d) £4500
e) £6500

4. An investor with £80,000 buys Moon Ltd shares when the mid-price is 25p (week 1). He takes £10,000 of profit out in week 2. In week 3 he reinvests this profit. How much does he have in week 4? (using the mid-price for all calculations)

a) £87,333
b) £144,000
c) £128,999
d) £151,499
e) £225,000

7. Soft Drink Sales

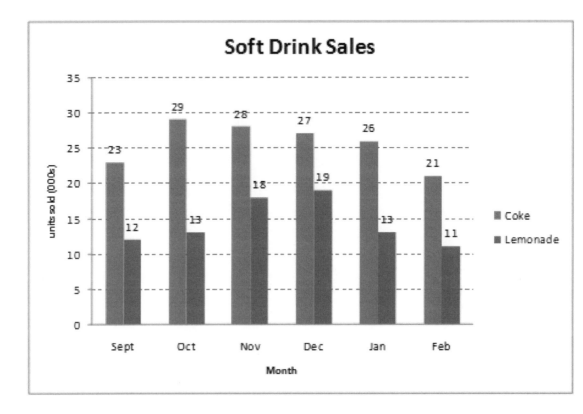

1. Which two months show the largest difference between the number of units of lemonade sold?

a) September and October
b) October and November
c) November and December
d) December and January
e) January and February

2. In October, what percentage of the total number of sales is attributable to Coke?

a) 13.6%
b) 15.1%
c) 31%
d) 69%
e) 75%

86

3. Which of the following showed the greatest sales?

a) Lemonade sales for December January and February
b) Lemonade sales for September October and November
c) Coke sales for January and February
d) Coke sales for September and October
e) Lemonade sales for September, January and February

4. In which month was the total sales greatest?

a) September
b) October
c) November
d) January
e) February

8. The Wedding Kitchen Company

Below are the charges made by the Wedding Kitchen Company for catering at a wedding:

Transport (per wedding)

Within 5 miles	5.1-10 miles	10.1 - 20 miles
£100	£150	£180

Staff (per night)

Chef	£200
Other Kitchen Staff	£300
Waiting Staff	£200

Menu (per cover)

Beef	£4.72
Lamb	£5.21
Vegetarian	£2.89

1. Alice and Raj are getting married and have invited 140 guests for one night. They estimate that about 10% will be vegetarian and the remainder will split

50/50 between beef and lamb. What will their estimated bill be for the menu alone?

a) £350.28
b) £528.39
c) £601.96
d) £666.05
e) £708.90

2. Alice and Raj can't decide between two different venues. One is 3 miles from the caterers, the other 17 miles. They hope to have the staff for Saturday night only. By choosing the closer venue, how many extra guests could they have without spending any more, assuming all the extra guests were to choose lamb?

a) 0
b) 8
c) 15
d) 16
e) None of the above

After getting all of the replies to their invites, the final numbers are:
Beef: 58 covers
Lamb: 62 covers
Vegetarian: 9 covers

3. They decided to go for the further venue in the end (17 miles from the caterer). What is their final bill going to be?
a) £1089.65
b) £1502.79
c) £1990.29
d) £2508.42
e) £3384.01

4. What would be the difference in price between a wedding with all 100 guests vegetarian, compared to a wedding with all 100 guests choosing lamb (assuming all other costs are the same)?

a) £211
b) £217
c) £232
d) £302
e) £521

9. Book Tables

The following bestselling book table is published in the newspaper:

Rank	Book	Copies sold (previous week)	Copies sold (total)	Rank Previous Week
1	The Crow	10,324	120,548	3
2	Loving Tenderness	9,089	352,429	2
3	Trains of Thought	5,437	1,003,420	1
4	The Crazed Maniac	3,392	3,392	-
5	Eating My Greens	3,254	77,432	6

1. Which book was released last week?

a) The Crow
b) Loving Tenderness
c) Trains of Thought
d) The Crazed Maniac
e) Eating My Greens

2. What was the total number of copies of Loving Tenderness that had been sold at the end of the previous week?

a) 243,786
b) 343,340
c) 352,429
d) 761,660
e) 997,983

3. By what percentage did sales of Trains of Thought increase from last week?

a) 0.542%
b) 0.545%
c) 0.549%
d) 5.42%
e) Can't say

4. The Crow was released 12 weeks ago. What was the average number of copies sold each week until a week ago?

a) 6, 548
b) 9, 899
c) 9, 998
d) 10,020
e) 10,324

10. Moon Limited

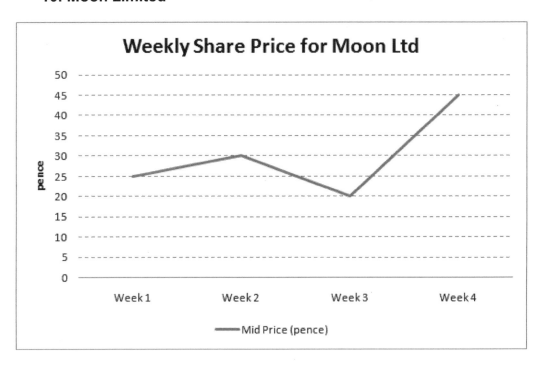

The mid price is calculated as halfway between the open price on the stock market at 8 a.m. on Monday morning and the close price for the week at 5 p.m. on Friday.

1. The mid-week share price in week 5 fell by 5%, what was the share price in week 5?

a) 40p
b) 42.75p
c) 42.86p
d) 47.37p

e) None of the above

2. A financial analyst has an extra week's worth of data to that shown (week 5). She calculates that the average mid price for weeks 1, 2, 3, 4 & 5 is 35 pence. What is the mid-week share price for week 5?

a) 24p
b) 31p
c) 35p
d) 55p
e) Can't say

3. By how much is the difference in Mid Price between weeks 1 and 4 greater than the difference in Mid Price between weeks 2 and 3?

a) 5p
b) 10p
c) 15p
d) 20p
e) 25p

4. Assume all investors buy and sell shares at the Mid Price. Given the following investment decisions, which investor achieves the greatest profit?

a) Investor A buys 1000 shares in week 1 and sells in week 2
b) Investor B buys 1000 shares in week 2 and sells in week 4
c) Investor C buys 500 shares in week 3 and sells in week 4
d) Investor D buys 500 shares in week 1 and sells in week 3
e) Investor E buys 500 shares in week 1 and sells in week 4

11. Motor Vehicle Sales

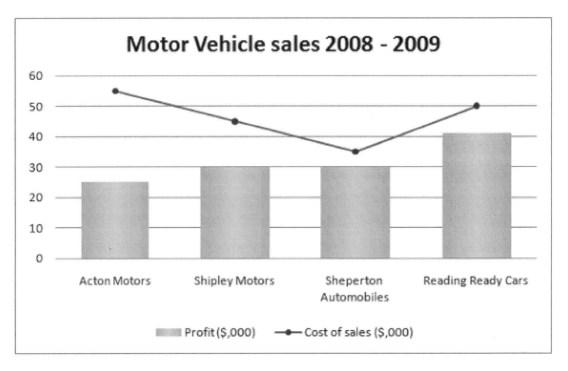

1. What is the mean cost of sales for all four companies?

a) $41,000
b) $30,000
c) $37,750
d) $46,250
e) $64,000

2. Which company had the largest turnover during the year?

a) Acton Motors
b) Shipley Motors
c) Sheperton Automobiles
d) Reading Ready Cars
e) Can't Say

3. What was the difference between the Company with the highest turnover and the company with the lowest turnover for the year?

a) $10,000
b) $15,000
c) $27,000
d) $35,000
e) $40,000

4. During 2010 each company is able to reduce its cost of sales by exactly $5,000. If the turnover for each company remains the same for 2010 which company would make the most profit?

a) Acton Motors
b) Shipley Motors
c) Sheperton Automobiles
d) Reading Ready Cars
e) Can't Say

12. Population statistics

Population statistics 1996

Location	Start of Year Population (millions)	Live Births per 1000 population during year	Deaths per 1000 population during year	% of population under 16 at year start	% of population aged over 65 at year start
Yorkshire	1.2	12.5	10.9	30	23
East Anglia	2.5	11.2	11.6	27	20
West Wales	0.5	14.5	12.6	25	36
London	3.5	9.6	9.8	24	15
Cornwall	0.8	9.5	11.8	16	42

1. Which region had the greatest number of people aged under 16 at the beginning of the year?

a) Cornwall
b) East Anglia
c) London
d) West Wales
e) Yorkshire

2. How many live births were there in Cornwall in 1996?

a) 6400
b) 6800
c) 7200
d) 7600
e) 8000

3. The death rate of those over 65 is 8% per year. How many people over 65, alive in Wales at the start of 1996, would die during the year?

a) 712
b) 2268
c) 2610
d) 6300
e) 10,865

4. Which region had the biggest growth in population in 1996? (Based only on birth and death rates)

a) Cornwall
b) East Anglia
c) London
d) West Wales
e) Yorkshire

13. Student Mess Budget

Budget for Student Mess 2008-9

Item	Percentage
Cereals	6
Confectionary	13
Newspapers	21
Cleaning services	12
Furnishings	23
Amenities	25
Total Value	£12,500

1. How much more of the budget is allocated to Furnishings, Amenities and Newspapers compared with all the other expenditures combines?

a) £3875
b) £4750
c) £7750
d) £8625
e) £9760

2. What combination of budgetary items would give a total expenditure of £4,375?

a) Cereals and Amenities
b) Cleaning Services and Furnishings
c) Confectionary and Amenities
d) Confectionary and Furnishings
e) Newspapers and Cleaning Services

3. Last year, the amount spent on newspapers was £500 less than this year and nothing was spent on cereals. The amounts spent on the other items was the same. What was the total budget last year?

a) £10750
b) £11250
c) £11750
d) £12000
e) £12250

4. How much of the budget is not spent on newspapers?

a) £10331
b) £2625
c) £6983
d) £9875
e) None of the above

14. Tax return

The following are the accounts for Moving.inc, a company that specialises in helping people relocate to foreign countries.

	Oct-Mar 2008	Apr-Sep 2008	Oct-Mar 2009	Apr-Sep 2009
No. of moves	28	43	39	62
Money In	£7000	£8500	£9750	£17050
Costs	£2950	£3110	£4120	£7085

Annual Cost Breakdown

Cost Type	Percentage of total costs
Insurance	12
Fuel	20
Vehicle acquisition and maintenance	38
Personnel	23
Other	7

1. The average price per move charged by the company was higher in one period than in the others. Which one was it?

a) Oct-Mar 2008
b) Apr-Sep 2008
c) Oct-Mar 2009
d) Apr-Sep 2009

2. In what period was the biggest profit per move made?

a) Oct-Mar 2008
b) Apr-Sep 2008
c) Oct-Mar 2009
d) Apr-Sep 2009

3. A new tax rule introduced in Oct-Mar 2009 meant that Insurance costs could no longer be deducted from tax. What was the extra cost to the company per month between April and September 2009 (6 month period)?

a) £108.90
b) £199.30
c) £341
d) £850.20
e) £141.70

4. After reviewing the costs for the period October 2008 - September 2009, the CEO decides to switch to a cheaper type of vehicle. Over the next year, he expects the move to cost the company £2100 less than was spent in the previous year on vehicle acquisition and maintenance. What does he expect the bill to be for vehicle maintenance and acquisition in 2009-2010?

a) £2157.90
b) £592.30
c) £8084
d) £4985
e) £4460.70

15. Timber Trading

Company	Annual Profit (£million)	Annual Turnover (£million)	Number of Employees
Redwood Timber	50	1500	2000
Balsa Inc.	30	125	1200
Oaktree exports	15	90	750
Hardwood Lumber Ltd	45	100	600
Canadian Timber	5	50	500

Profit = Turnover - Costs

1. An investor is looking to invest in one of the companies. Which company has the highest annual profit per employee?

a) Redwood Timber
b) Balsa Inc.
c) Oaktree Exports
d) Hardwood Lumber Ltd
e) Canadian Timber

2. What was the percentage of turnover was profit for Balsa Inc.?

a) 4.17%
b) 19%
c) 24%
d) 25%
e) 50%

3. Which company makes the least percentage of profit from turnover?

a) Redwood Timber
b) Balsa Inc.
c) Oaktree Exports
d) Hardwood Lumber Ltd
e) Canadian Timber

4. Canadian Timber pays its employees on average £30,000 per year. What proportion of costs do wages make up?

a) 30%
b) 33.3%
c) 27%
d) 7.5%
e) 3.3%

16. Unit Sales

Below is a pie chart showing the number of sales for 5 different units of a company:

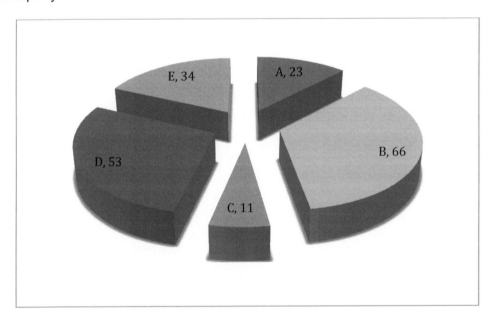

1. What were the total sales for all units?

a) 176
b) 164
c) 187
d) 210
e) 221

2. What percentage of total sales came from Unit D?

a) 12%
b) 18%
c) 28%
d) 35%
e) 40%

3. How much greater was the percentage of sales from Units A and B combined compared to Units C and E combined?

a) 4%
b) 14%
c) 24%
d) 28%
e) 56%

4. What percentage of total sales came from units A, C and E ?

a) 28%
b) 36%
c) 57%
d) 63%
e) None of the above

17. Yoghurt

The following is the information given on the back of your yoghurt pack at home:

	Per 125g serving	% daily allowance
Energy (KJ)	518	-
Energy (Kcal)	123	6
Protein (g)	4.4	10
Carbohydrate (g)	17.3	8
Fat (g)	4.0	6
Fibre (g)	0.3	1
Sodium (g)	0.1	3

1. How many kilojoules are there in a kilocalorie?

a) 0.24
b) 5.18
c) 4.2
d) 1.23
e) 8

2. To gain my total daily energy allowance, how many whole yoghurts (of 125g) would I need to eat?

a) 12
b) 16
c) 17
d) 22
e) 33

3. I eat two yoghurts and then a packet of crisps which contains 23% of my daily allowance of sodium. How many grams of sodium have I eaten?

a) 0.43g
b) 0.87g
c) 0.97g
d) 1.08g
e) 14.68g

4. The total calorific content of the food is measured by adding together the calories in the protein, fat and carbohydrate. Carbohydrate provides 4 Kcal per g, fat 9 Kcal per g. How many calories per gram of protein are there, to the nearest Kcal?

100

a) 2
b) 3
c) 4
d) 5
e) 10

18: Household Energy Suppliers

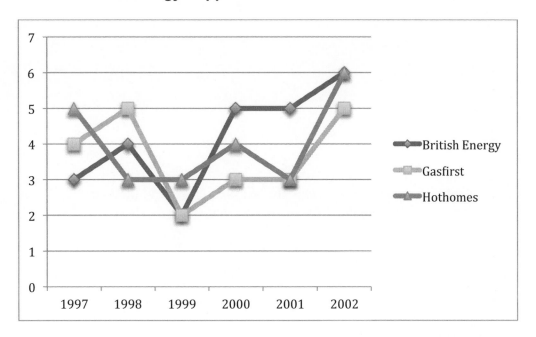

The chart shows the percentage rise in the average bill each year between 1997 and 2002 (inclusive) for three different companies. The figures given are for the rise that has occurred over the year, for example, the average bill for Hothomes increased 4% over the year 2000.

In 1996, the average annual bill for British Energy was £300, Gasfirst was £280 and Hothomes was £320.

1. What was the average percentage rise in a bill for British Energy between 1997 and 2000 inclusive?

a) 9.3%

b) 14%
c) 14.7%
d) 15%
e) 17%

2. What was the average bill for a customer of Gasfirst at the start of 1999?

a) £291
b) £291.20
c) £294
d) £305.76
e) £311.88

3. What was the average rise per year over the 6 year period for Hothomes?

a) 3.66%
b) 4%
c) 4.16%
d) 4.28%
e) 5%

4. At the end of 2001 Hothomes added an extra £33 to the bill of each customer in the South West region. What was the average total bill at the end of that year for Hothomes customers there?

a) £381.84
b) £404.75
c) £409.00
d) £414.84
e) £437.75

Quantitative Reasoning Practice Question Answers

1. Travelling to Chamonix

1. e) 5 hrs 42 minutes
1 hr 38 (car) + 90 (airport) + 1 hr 15 (flight) + 30 (waiting for train) + 49 (train) = 342 minutes = 5 hrs 42 minutes

2. c) 39.8 miles
Car: Number of miles per gallon = 74.6 miles / (8.95 / 6.26) = 52.2 mpg (or: 46.7 / (5.6 / 6.26) = 52.2)
Bus: Miles per gallon = 20 x (1000 / 1609) = 12.4 mpg
52.2 - 12.4 = 39.8 extra miles per gallon

This is quite a complex calculation of the time allowed. You can quickly narrow down the answer to 39.8 by excluding the other answers which are not in the correct ball park – in this case all of the other options.

3. d) £86.45
The cheapest way is obviously via Cardiff and then on the train:
£8.95 + £65 + (15/1.2) = £86.45, or 103.7 Euros

4. b) 828.38 miles
3085km can quickly be excluded as from eye-balling the figures, the answer should be around 1200-1500 km or 800-900 miles
Total distance is less if travelling from Bristol, so only this calculation need be made:
(46.7 miles x 1609) + (730.9 miles x 1609) + (81.7 x 1000) = total distance in metres = 1332858.4 metres, or **828.38 miles**
Alternatively, (81.7 x 1000) / 1609 = 50.78 miles
46.7 + 730.9 + 50.78 = **828.38 miles**

2. Cycling Speed

1. e) 50km
During leg 1 she travels 15 x 1 = 15 km
During leg 2 she travels 5 x 1 = 5 km
During leg 3 she travels 20 x 1.5 = 30 km
Total distance = 50km

2. e) 70km

During leg 1 she travels 15 x 1 = 15 km
During leg 2 she travels 5 x 1 = 5 km
During leg 3 she travels 20 x 2 = 40 km
During leg 4 she travels 10 x 1 = 10 km
Total distance = 70km

3. b) 5km/h faster

She takes 1 hour to travel the distance between 1 and 2 hours into her journey. You wish to reduce the total time taken by 0.5 hours. Therefore, she must complete this leg in half the time; which she can achieve by doubling her speed. She should therefore travel 5km per hour faster. Important note: read the question carefully - it asks you how much faster (5km/h), rather than how fast (10km/h).

4. c) 4 hours and 25 minutes

Cyclist A travels 15km (15 / 1) in 1 hour. Cyclist B travels this distance in (15/20) = 0.75 hours
Cyclist A travels 10km (10 / 1) in 1 hour. Cyclist B travels this distance in (10/15) = 0.67 hours
The other sections of the journey are covered in the same time at the same speed.
Therefore the time taken is 0.75 + 1 + 2 + 0.67 = 4.42 hours
This is the same as 4 hours and 25 minutes.

3. Dunvoor Ferry Timetable

1. c) 38 miles/hour

95 minutes = 95/60 = 1.58333 hours
A single crossing is 120/2 = 60 miles
Speed = distance / time = 60 miles / 1.58333 = 38 miles per hour

2. d) 1200

The ferry departs at 08 45 and arrives in Logan point at 10 20 (95 minutes crossing time). It makes the required wait until 11:35 (1 hour and 15 minutes) and is therefore ready for the next return crossing which is 12:00 (having just missed the 11:30).

3. e) None of the above

If he wishes to return at 09:00, following a 1 hour and 15 minute wait, the latest he must arrive in Logan point is 07:45. He must therefore leave 95 minutes before this, at 0610. The answer is 'None of the above'

4. c) 0800
He must arrive by 0950
95 minutes before 0950 is 0815
The last ferry before 0815 is at 0800

4. Fence Painting

1. a) 0.71 m^2
Area of a circle = Pi x r^2
= 3.14159 x (0.3 x 0.3)
= 0.2827
But these are in fact semi-circles so halve the value and multiply by the number of panels, so
(0.2827 / 2) x 5 = 0.71m^2 (2 decimal places)

2. d) 2.70m
The area of one panel can be calculated as width * height. As we know the top of the panel is decorated by a perfect semi-circle it's width must be double the radius or 0.6m. So the area of one panel is
= 0.9 x 0.6
= 0.54 m^2
Thus the total area is 0.54 x 5 (the number of panels)
= 2.70 m^2

3. a) 3.41 m^2
Total area of semi-circular panelling (from question 1)
= 0.71 m^2
Total area of main panelling (from question 2)
= 2.7 m^2
Therefore total area is given by
= 2.7 + 0.71
= 3.41 m^2

4. d) 0.99L
Total area to paint is 3.41m^2.
(3.41 / 10) x 100% = 34.1% of the pot used. She will have 65.9% of the tin remaining.
(65.9 x 1.5L) / 100 = 0.99L remaining

5. Flying

1. c) 3 hrs 25 mins
This is simply the difference between the arrival times at Delhi:
0330 - 0005 = 3 hours and 25 minutes

2. b) 1450 miles

Flying time:

London - Vienna = 09.15 - 12.40, minus 1 hour time difference = 2 hrs 25 minutes

2 hrs 25 minutes = 145 minutes

600mph / 60 = 10 miles per minute

10 x 145 = 1450 miles

3. c) 9 hrs 35 mins

London to Abu Dhabi = 0915 - 1920 = 10 hours and 5 minutes

minus 4 hours = 6 hours and 5 minutes

Abu Dhabi to Delhi is 2230 - 0330 = 5 hours

minus 1 and a half hours = 3 hours and 30 minutes

add 6:05 and 3:30 = 9 hours and 35 minutes

4. d) 9.4p/mile

Total Flying Time (from previous question) is 9 hours 35 minutes

= 575 minutes, at 10 miles per minute = 5750 miles from London to Abu Dhabi

543.37 / 5750 miles = £0.094 = 9.4 pence/mile

6. Moon Limited

1. c) £15.00

100 shares @ 30p in week 2 = £30 of shares. The percentage appreciation between weeks 2 and 4 is from 30p to 45p = a 50% increase. Therefore the new value of the shares at the end of week 4 is (1 + 0.5) x £30 = £45 which equates to a £15 profit!

2. b) £40,500

The initial investment will have gone up 50% three times over the 6 weeks. The calculation required is therefore 12000 x 1.5 x 1.5 x 1.5 = £40,500

3. b) £1500

£5000 x 20/25 = amount left at week 3 = £4000

£4000 / 2 = £2000

£2000 x 45/20 = increase in value of the remainder by week 4 = £4500

£4500 + £2000 = £6500

Therefore his profit is £1500

4. d) £151,499

Initial investment was £80,000

£80,000 x 30/25 = £96,000 in week 2

£10,000 profit withdrawn = £86,000

Week 3 Total = £86,000 x 20/30 = £57,333
£57,333 + £10,000 reinvested = £67,333
Week 4 Total: £67,333 x 45/20 = £151,499

7. Soft Drink Sales

1. d) December and January
The biggest difference is between December and January (6,000 units) that is (19,000 - 13,000 on the chart)

2. d) 69%
For October the total number of sales is 29 + 13 = 42. Therefore the proportion of Coke sales is 100 x 29/42 = 69%

3. d) Coke sales for September and October
Lemonade sales for December January and February:
19 + 13 + 11 = 43
Lemonade sales for September October and November:
12 + 13 + 18 = 43
Coke sales for January and February:
26 + 21 = 47
Coke sales for September and October:
23 + 29 = 52
Lemonade sales for September, January and February:
12 + 13 + 11 = 36

4. c) November

8. The Wedding Kitchen Company

1. d) £666.05
10% of 140 = 14 vegetarians
(140-14)/2 = the number of covers for both beef and lamb = 63 each
14 x 2.89 = 40.46
63 x 5.21 = 328.23
63 x 4.72 = 297.36
40.46 + 328.23 + 297.36 = £666.05

2. c) 15
By choosing the closer venue, the couple will save £80.
£80 / £5.21 = 15.35 = 15 extra guests

3. b) £1502.79
Travel: £180

Staff = £200 + £300 + £200 = £700
58 x £4.72 = £273.76
62 x £ 5.21 = £323.02
9 x £2.89 = £26.01
Total = 180 + 708 + 273.76 + 323.02 + 26.01 = **£1502.79**

4. c) £232
If all other costs remain the same, the difference in price is:
100 x 5.21 = £521
100 x 2.89 = £289
£521 - £289 = £232

9. Book Tables

1. d) The Crazed Maniac
This book did not have a rank last week. The total sales and sales over the last week are the same.

2. b) 343,340
352,429 - 9,089 = 343,340

3. b) 0.545%
At the end of last week, total number of sales of Trains of Thought were:
1,003,420 - 5,437 = 997,983
Subsequently, 5,437 copies were sold.
The percentage increase is 5,437 / 997,983 x 100 = 0.545 %

4. d) 10,020
120,548 – 10,324 = 110,224
110,224 / 11 = 10,020 copies

Set 2

10. Moon Limited

1. b) 42.75p
45 x (1 - 0.05) = 42.75p

2. d) 55p
35p x 5 weeks = 175p as the total price over the period. 175p - 25p - 30p - 20p - 45p (from the graph) = 55p

3. b) 10p
(45p - 25p) - (30p - 20p) = 10p

4. b) Investor B
Investor A generates (30 - 25) * 1000 = 5,000 pence profit
Investor B generates (45 - 30) * 1000 = 15,000 pence profit
Investor C generates (45 - 20) * 500 = 12,500 pence profit
Investor D generates (20 - 25) * 500 = - 2,500 pence profit
Investor E generates (45 - 25) * 500 = 10,000 pence profit

11. Motor Vehicle Sales

1. d) $46,250
From the graph :
($1000 x (55 + 45 + 35 + 50)) / 4 = $46,250

2. d) Reading Ready Cars
Turnover = $42,000 + $50,000 = $92,000

3. c) $27,000
Reading Ready Cars ($92,000 turnover) - Sheperton Automobiles ($65,000 turnover)

4. d) Reading Ready Cars
The trick here is to realise that this is a straight linear transformation.
The long way is to evaluate the turnover for 2008 - 2009 then recalculate the profit for the subsequent year by reducing the cost of sales for $5,000 with the equation given. However this is not necessary.
If the cost of sales is reduced by $5,000 but the turnover remains the same the profit will rise by $5,000 for each Company. Therefore Reading Ready cars will make the most profit as it did the previous year.

12. Population statistics

1. c) London
1.2 x 30% = 0.36 million (Yorkshire)
2.5 x 27% = 0.675 million (East Anglia)
0.5 x 25% = 0.125 million (West Wales)
3.5 x 24% = 0.84 million (London)
0.8 x 16% = 0.128 million (Cornwall)

2. d) 7600
In Cornwall, the population is 0.8 million, or 800,000
800,000 / 1000 = 800
800 x 9.5 = 7600

3. b) 2268
36/100 x 0.5 million = 0.18 million, or 180,000 people over 65 in Wales at year start. There were 12.6 deaths per 1000 over the year:
(180,000 / 1000) x 12.6 = 2268

4. e) Yorkshire
You can tell this simply by looking at the data:
East Anglia, London and Cornwall had higher death rates than live birth rates. Therefore, based only on these figures, populations here would have decreased. Yorkshire and Wales both had higher numbers of live births than deaths. In Yorkshire, the starting population was bigger and the net % increase was more than in Wales.

13. Student Mess Budget

1. b) £4750
Total percentage for furnishings, amenities and newspapers: 25% + 23% + 21% = 69%,
Other expenditures = 1 00% - 69% = 31%
Difference = 69% - 31% = 38%
Therefore amount = 38% x £12,500 = £4,750

2. b) Cleaning Services and Furnishings
£4,375 / £12,500 = 35% of the budget. The only two items that when combined would take a 35% stake are Cleaning Services + Furnishings.

3. b) £11250
6% of £12500 is £750
Last year, the total budget was £12500 - £750 - £500 = £11250

4. d) £9875
100% - 21% (newspapers) = 79%
£12,500 x 79/100 = £9,875

14. Tax return

1. d) Apr-Sep 2009
In the first 3 periods, the average charge per move was £250
In Apr-Sep 2009 the charge was £17050 / 62 = £275

2. d) Apr-Sep 2009
Oct-Mar 2008 Profit per move was: (£7000 - £2950)/28 = £144.64

110

Apr-Sep 2008 Profit per move was: (£8500 - £3110) / 34 = £158.53
Oct-Mar 2009 Profit per move was: (£9750 - £4120) / 39 = £144.36
Apr-Sep 2009 (£17050 - £7085) / 62 = £160.73

3. e) £141.70
£7085 x 0.12 = £850.20
850.20 / 6 = £141.70

4. a) £2157.90
In Oct 2008- Sept 2009, costs of vehicle acquisition and maintenance were :
0.38 x £(4120 + 7085) = £4257.90
He expects to save £2100 on the bill for vehicles in 2009 - 2010, so: £4257.90 -
£2100 = **£2157.90**

15. Timber Trading

1. d) Hardwood Lumber Ltd
You can tell this simply by looking at the data. Hardwood Lumber Ltd has
relatively few employees and one of the highest annual profits.
45,000,000 / 600 = £75,000 per employee

2. c) 24%
30/125 x 100 = 24%

3. a) Redwood Timber
This does not require a calculation - it can be clearly seen that 50/1500 is lower
than any of the other percentages of profit.

4. b) 33.3%
£30,000 x 500 = £15 million
Costs were £45 million
15/45 million = 33.3%

16. Unit Sales

1. c) 187
66 + 11 + 53 + 34 + 23 = 187

2. c) 28%
100 x 53 / (53 + 11 + 66 + 23 + 34) = 28.3%

3. c) 24%
Total sales for all units: 23 + 66 + 11 + 53 + 34 = 187
Percentage of sales from A and B combined:

100 x (23 + 66) / 187 = 24%
Therefore 48% - 24% = 24% difference

4. b) 36%
(23 + 11 + 34) / 187 = 0.36 = 36%

17. Yoghurt

1. c) 4.2
518 / 123 = 4.2 KJ/Kcal

2. c) 17
125g provides 6% of daily allowance, therefore:
100% / 6% = 16.6 = 17 yoghurts

3. c) 0.97g
0.1g is 3% of daily allowance. Therefore 100% is (0.1 / 3) x 100 = 3.33g
(3.33 x 23) / 100 = Sodium in the packet of crisps = 0.77g
0.77 + 0.1 + 0.1 = 0.97g

4. c) 4
123 - (4 x 17.3) - (9 x 4.0) = Number of Kcal provided by 4.4g protein = 17.8
17.8 / 4.4 = 4Kcal/g protein

18: Household Energy Suppliers

1. c) This question requires cumulative average percentage rises to be calculated.
so: 1 x 1.03 x 1.04 x 1.02 x 1.05 = 1.147 = **14.7%**

2. d)
£280 x 1.04 x 1.05 = £305.76

3. b)
5 + 3 + 3 + 4 + 3 + 6 = 24
24 / 6 = average 4% rise over the 6 years

4. d)
£320 x 1.05 x 1.03 x 1.03 x 1.04 x 1.03 = £381.84
£381.84 + £33 = £414.84

Chapter 3

Abstract Reasoning

Abstract Reasoning

UKCAT says 'Abstract reasoning assesses your ability to identify patterns amongst abstract shapes where irrelevant and distracting material may lead to incorrect conclusions. The test therefore measures your ability to change track, critically evaluate and generate hypotheses and requires you to query judgements as you go along.'

What is it?

There are 4 types of question:

1) You are presented with two sets of six groups of shapes that are related to each other in some way. You are asked to identify the pattern that links the shape sets and decide whether further shape groups fit with either, or neither, of the sets.
2) You will be asked for the next shape in a series of shapes.
3) You are given a statement involving a group of shapes and asked to decide which shape completes the statement.
4) You will be asked which of a number of shapes belongs to sets 'group A' or 'group B'.

You are given 14 minutes to read the instructions and answer 55 questions. This allows you **14 seconds per question**. In practice, you will probably spend 30-40 seconds identifying the theme and then answer the questions quickly.

This is perhaps the section of the exam that requires the most practice. The UKCAT format used asks you to identify themes within two different sets of shapes and then decide whether separate shape sets fit with set A, set B or neither (none). Usually, the common theme linking all the patterns in set A will be similar to the common theme linking all the patterns in set B. For example, in set A, all the patterns may contain a black circle in the top right corner. In set B, all the patterns may contain a black square in the bottom left corner. There will usually be other shapes of varying colours and sizes in the boxes that are placed randomly and act as 'distractors'. Identifying the linking theme can be complex and it helps to have a structured approach.

Look at the **simplest** patterns first. These still have something in common with the other patterns but there are fewer distractors.

Think about commonly used 'themes':

- **Check the numbers and types of shapes in each pattern**
- **Check the shading and the outline**
- **Look at the numbers and angles of the sides and overlaps**
- **Look for relationships between the shapes such as position or symmetry**
- **Look at the gaps and 'what is not there'**
- **Remember that there may be two linked patterns involved, for example each set may contain an odd number of shapes *and* at least one of them is shaded**
- **If you are unable to identify a theme, look at the other questions relating to the set, as this might provide a clue**

Why is Abstract Reasoning in the exam?

This part of the exam 'measures your ability to change track, critically evaluate and generate hypotheses and query your judgements as you go along'. Thinking critically and reflectively is a key component of professional life - you should always be asking yourself if something can be done or explained in a better way. You must be prepared to assess and change your practice if you find it can. In medicine, you will be expected to demonstrate this practice annually at an 'appraisal'. The examiner's theory is that the puzzles in this part of the test try to check for this skill by requiring you to form hypotheses about how the patterns are linked and then check it. If you find any reason to doubt your hypothesis you then have to develop a new hypothesis and check that.

Worked Examples

See if you can identify the theme in the following shape sets:

Think particularly about shape type, position, shading and number.

Set A

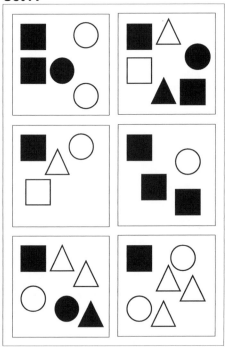

Type: Three different shapes are present. Not all shapes are present in each box.

Shading: Number shaded and shapes shaded varies in each box

Number: The total number of shapes varies in each box

Position: There is a shaded square in the top left corner. All other shape positions appear to be random.

The linking 'theme' is that 'There is a shaded square in the top left hand corner of each box'.

Once you have identified a possible theme, you should be able to identify a similar theme in set B:

116

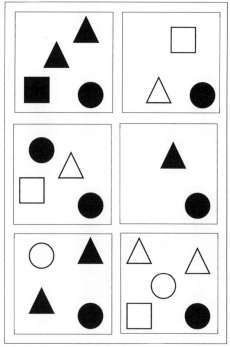

Again, there are three different types of shapes present and not all are present in each box. Shading and number of shapes is variable. There is however a shaded circle in the bottom right corner of each box. This confirms the 'theme'.

Hint: Look at the boxes with the least amount of information first. These contain fewer distractors and still have the characteristics to belong to the set.

Your task to then decide which set the following shape boxes belongs to becomes easy:

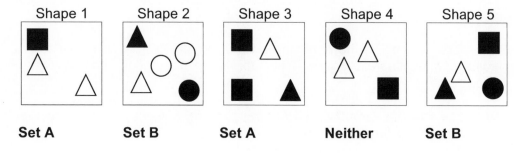

Adding complexity:

Set A

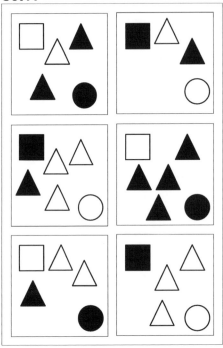

Type: Three different shapes are present and all are present in each box.

Shading: The number shaded in each box is variable

Number: There is one square and one circle in each box. There is a variable number of triangles in each box.

Position: There is a square in the top left hand corner and a circle in the bottom right hand corner of each square.

Added complexity: If the square is shaded, the circle is not. If the circle is shaded, the square is not.

(Remember to check if the shading and number of triangles is linked to the shading of the square or circle. Both appear to be random and these are 'distractors').

Hint: Once you have identified a linking pattern, always check for further linked patterns or 'added complexity'.

118

Set B

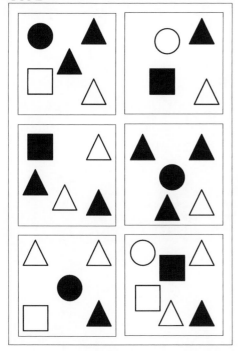

A similar pattern can be seen in Set B, the linking theme is that there is a triangle in the bottom right hand corner of each box. If that triangle is shaded there is a non-shaded triangle in the top right corner. If the triangle is not shaded, the triangle in the top right corner is shaded.

Once you have identified the theme(s), deciding which set the following shape boxes belong to is easy:

Shape 1 Shape 2 Shape 3 Shape 4 Shape 5

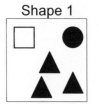 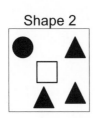 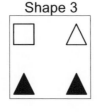 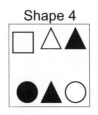 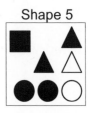

Answer:
Shape 1: Neither
Shape 2: Neither
Shape 3: Set B

119

Shape 4: Neither
Shape 5: Set A
Examples of other 'themes':

Number of lines (distractor: make shapes of a man symbol)
Rotation
Forming shapes
Number of shapes with 'shaded counting twice'

Other Abstract Reasoning Questions

You may be asked to select the next shape set in a series:

Which figure completes the series?

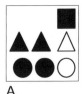 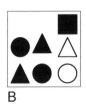 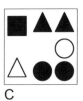 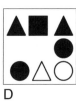

A   B   C   D

Answer: A

The three circles and the white triangle and rotating in an anti-clockwise manner. The square and black triangles are arranged randomly and are distractors.

120

You may be asked to identify how two shape sets relate to each other and deduce which shape set is related to a second in a similar way:

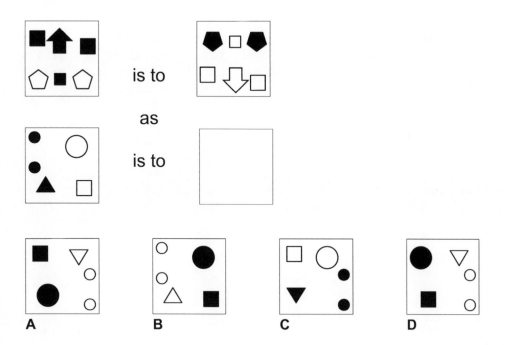

is to

as

is to

A   B   C   D

Answer: A

All the shapes have been rotated 180 degrees and the shading is the opposite. The same has happened in set A.

Abstract Reasoning Exercise

Take 1 minute to read these instructions.

You will be presented with two sets of shapes - 'set A' and 'set B'. Shapes in set A are all related to each other in some way. Shapes in set B are all related to each other in some way. Determine how the shapes within each set are related. You will be given 5 'test shapes' and must decide whether they should be in 'set A', 'set B' or 'Neither' ('None').

There is another type of question that involves choosing the correct shape to complete the sequence.

You have 3 and a 1/2 minutes to answer 21 questions. Try and answer all the questions. There is no negative marking.

Shape Set 1

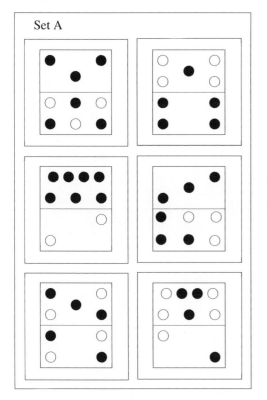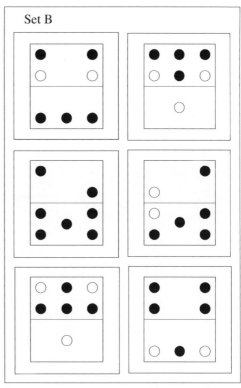

For each of the shapes below, decide whether they belong to Set A, Set B or neither

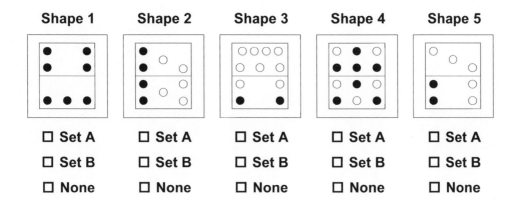

Shape 1	Shape 2	Shape 3	Shape 4	Shape 5
☐ Set A	☐ Set A	☐ Set A	☐ Set A	☐ Set A
☐ Set B	☐ Set B	☐ Set B	☐ Set B	☐ Set B
☐ None	☐ None	☐ None	☐ None	☐ None

Shape set 2

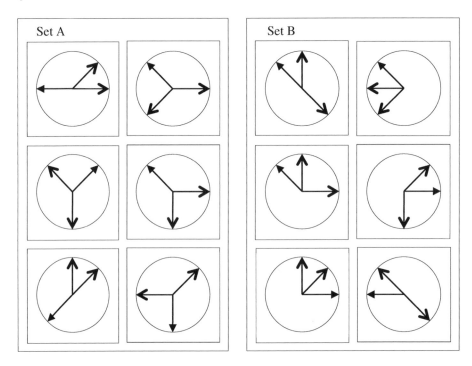

For each of the shapes below, decide whether they belong to Set A, Set B or neither

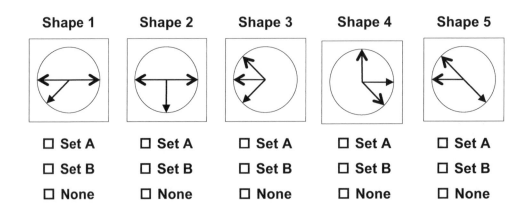

Shape 1	Shape 2	Shape 3	Shape 4	Shape 5
☐ Set A	☐ Set A	☐ Set A	☐ Set A	☐ Set A
☐ Set B	☐ Set B	☐ Set B	☐ Set B	☐ Set B
☐ None	☐ None	☐ None	☐ None	☐ None

Shape Set 3

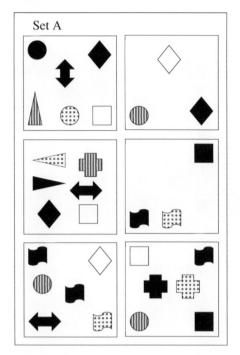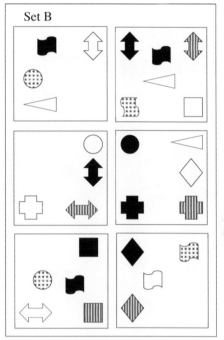

For each of the shapes below, decide whether they belong to Set A, Set B or neither

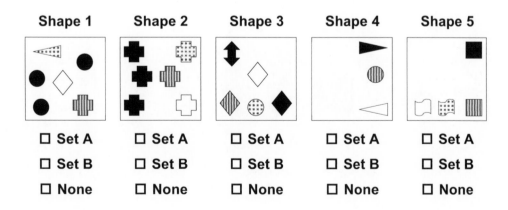

Shape 1	Shape 2	Shape 3	Shape 4	Shape 5
☐ Set A	☐ Set A	☐ Set A	☐ Set A	☐ Set A
☐ Set B	☐ Set B	☐ Set B	☐ Set B	☐ Set B
☐ None	☐ None	☐ None	☐ None	☐ None

Shape Set 4

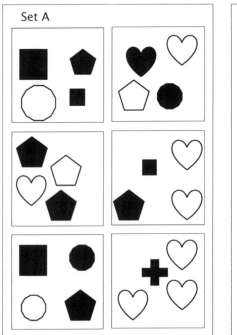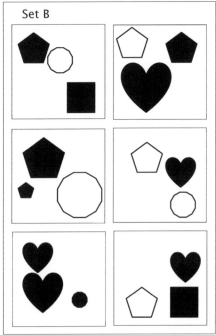

For each of the shapes below, decide whether they belong to Set A, Set B or neither

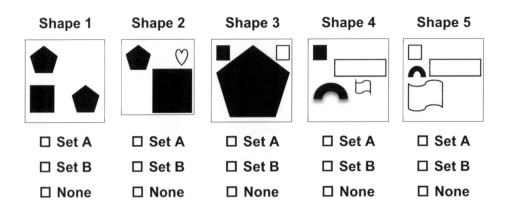

Shape 1	Shape 2	Shape 3	Shape 4	Shape 5
☐ Set A	☐ Set A	☐ Set A	☐ Set A	☐ Set A
☐ Set B	☐ Set B	☐ Set B	☐ Set B	☐ Set B
☐ None	☐ None	☐ None	☐ None	☐ None

Question 5

The following shapes are arranged in order.

 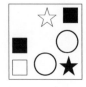 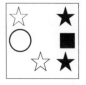

Which of the following comes next?

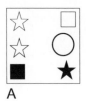 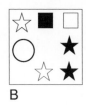 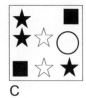 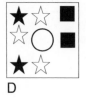

A   B   C   D

Answers

Shape Set 1

In Set A, the total number of spots is 9. There is an even number of spots in the lower half.

In Set B, the total number of spots is 7. There is an odd number of spots in the lower half.

The shading in both sets is irrelevant.

Shape 1: Set B
Shape 2: None
Shape 3: None
Shape 4: None
Shape 5: None

Shape Set 2

In set A the angle between the shaded and both non-shaded arrows is 90 degrees, 180 degrees or 135 degrees.

In set B the angle between the two non-shaded arrows is 30 degrees, 60 degrees or 120 degrees.

Shape 1: None
Shape 2: Set A
Shape 3: Set B
Shape 4: Set B
Shape 5: None

Shape Set 3

Set A contains 3 black shapes, one dotted shape the same as one of the black shapes, one stripe shape and one white shape.

Set B contains 2 black shapes, one striped shape the same as one of the black shapes, one dotted and two white shapes.

Shape 1: None
Shape 2: Set A
Shape 3: None
Shape 4: None
Shape 5: Set B

Shape Set 4

Set A contains four shapes.
Set B contains three shapes.

The shading and type of shape are distractors.

Shape 1: Set B
Shape 2: Set B
Shape 3: Set B
Shape 4: Set A
Shape 5: Set A

Question 5

The number of stars in each box increases by 1. The extra star is alternately a shaded and then a non-shaded star. The answer is therefore C. The squares and circle are distractors.

Abstract Reasoning Practice Questions

Depending on how many shape sets you are going to do, allow yourself the following time:

1 set: 70 seconds
2 sets: 2 minutes 20 seconds
5 sets: 5 minutes 50 seconds
10 sets: 11 minutes 40 seconds
11 sets: 13 minutes

Shape Set 1

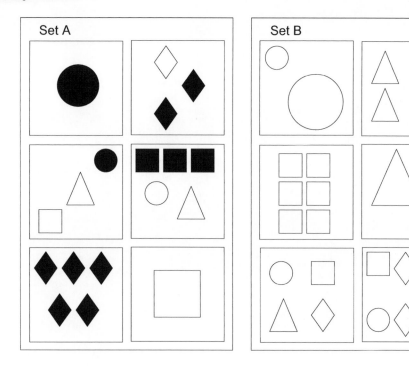

For each of the shapes below, decide whether they belong to Set A, Set B or Neither.

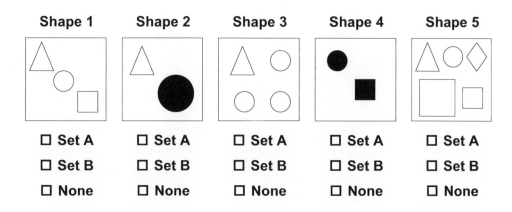

Shape 1	Shape 2	Shape 3	Shape 4	Shape 5
☐ Set A	☐ Set A	☐ Set A	☐ Set A	☐ Set A
☐ Set B	☐ Set B	☐ Set B	☐ Set B	☐ Set B
☐ None	☐ None	☐ None	☐ None	☐ None

131

Shape Set 2

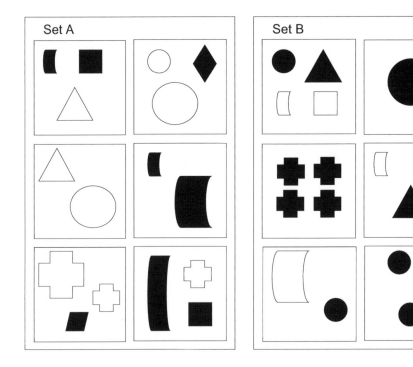

For each of the shapes below, decide whether they belong to Set A, Set B or Neither.

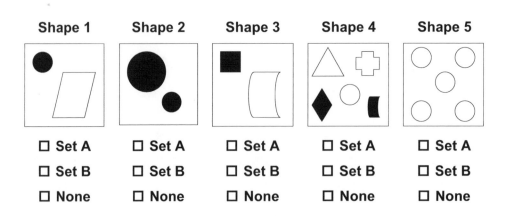

Shape Set 3

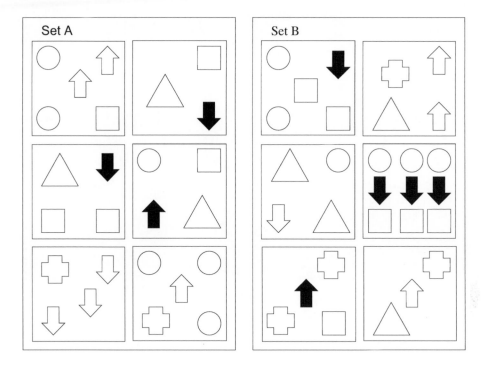

For each of the shapes below, decide whether they belong to Set A, Set B or Neither

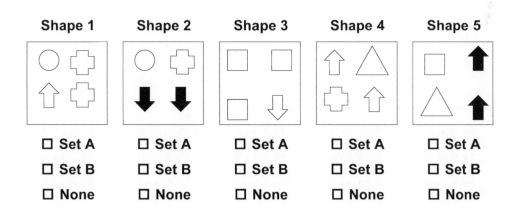

Shape 1	Shape 2	Shape 3	Shape 4	Shape 5
☐ Set A	☐ Set A	☐ Set A	☐ Set A	☐ Set A
☐ Set B	☐ Set B	☐ Set B	☐ Set B	☐ Set B
☐ None	☐ None	☐ None	☐ None	☐ None

Shape Set 4

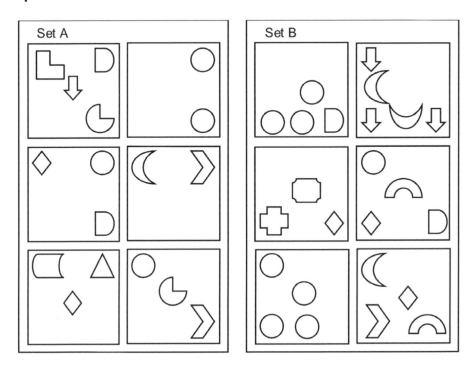

For each of the shapes below, decide whether they belong to Set A, Set B or Neither

Shape 1	Shape 2	Shape 3	Shape 4	Shape 5

☐ Set A   ☐ Set A   ☐ Set A   ☐ Set A   ☐ Set A

☐ Set B   ☐ Set B   ☐ Set B   ☐ Set B   ☐ Set B

☐ None   ☐ None   ☐ None   ☐ None   ☐ None

Shape Set 5

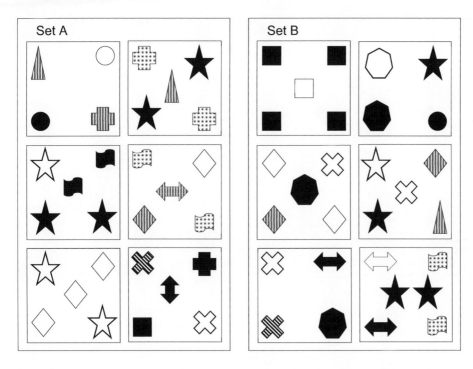

For each of the shapes below, decide whether they belong to Set A, Set B or Neither

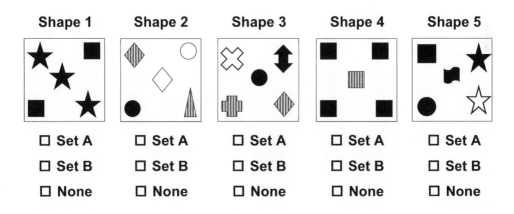

Shape Set 6

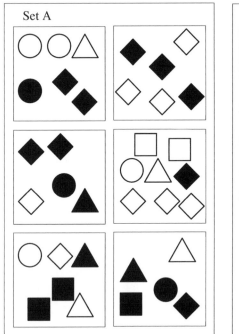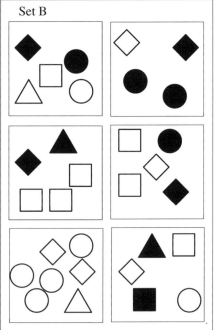

For each of the shapes below, decide whether they belong to Set A, Set B or Neither

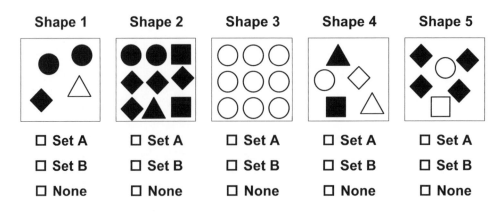

Shape 1	Shape 2	Shape 3	Shape 4	Shape 5
☐ Set A	☐ Set A	☐ Set A	☐ Set A	☐ Set A
☐ Set B	☐ Set B	☐ Set B	☐ Set B	☐ Set B
☐ None	☐ None	☐ None	☐ None	☐ None

Shape Set 7

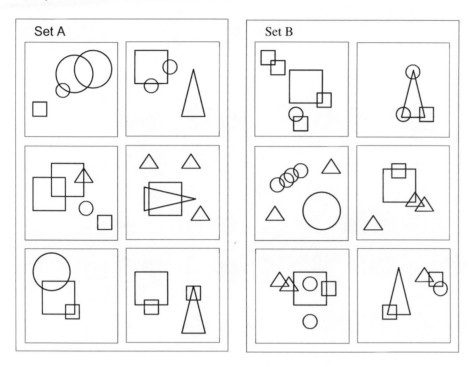

For each of the shapes below, decide whether they belong to Set A, Set B or Neither

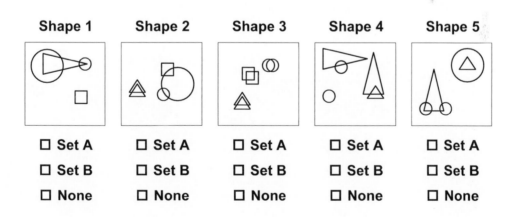

Shape 1	Shape 2	Shape 3	Shape 4	Shape 5
☐ Set A	☐ Set A	☐ Set A	☐ Set A	☐ Set A
☐ Set B	☐ Set B	☐ Set B	☐ Set B	☐ Set B
☐ None	☐ None	☐ None	☐ None	☐ None

137

Shape Set 8

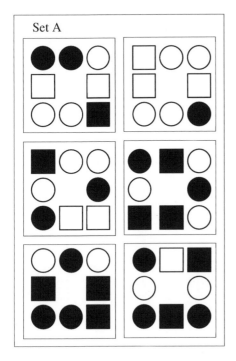 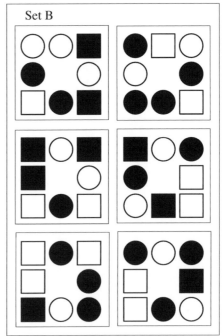

For each of the shapes below, decide whether they belong to Set A, Set B or Neither

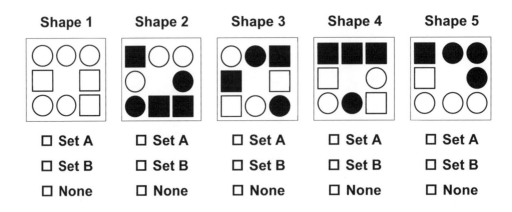

Shape 1	Shape 2	Shape 3	Shape 4	Shape 5
☐ Set A	☐ Set A	☐ Set A	☐ Set A	☐ Set A
☐ Set B	☐ Set B	☐ Set B	☐ Set B	☐ Set B
☐ None	☐ None	☐ None	☐ None	☐ None

138

Shape Set 9

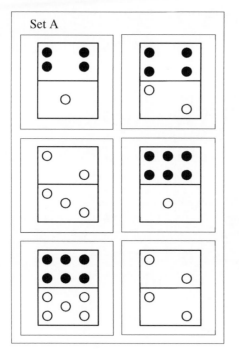

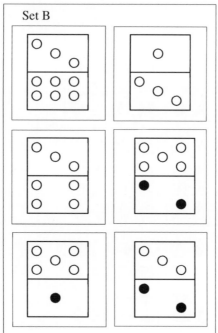

For each of the shapes below, decide whether they belong to Set A, Set B or Neither

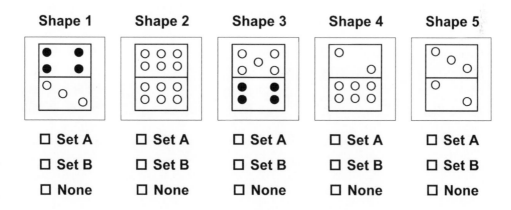

Shape 1	Shape 2	Shape 3	Shape 4	Shape 5
☐ Set A	☐ Set A	☐ Set A	☐ Set A	☐ Set A
☐ Set B	☐ Set B	☐ Set B	☐ Set B	☐ Set B
☐ None	☐ None	☐ None	☐ None	☐ None

Shape Set 10

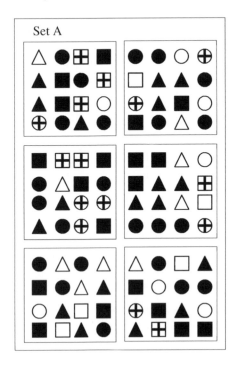

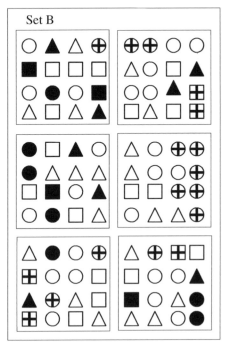

For each of the shapes below, decide whether they belong to Set A, Set B or Neither

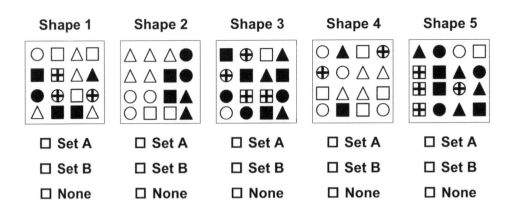

Shape 1	Shape 2	Shape 3	Shape 4	Shape 5
☐ Set A	☐ Set A	☐ Set A	☐ Set A	☐ Set A
☐ Set B	☐ Set B	☐ Set B	☐ Set B	☐ Set B
☐ None	☐ None	☐ None	☐ None	☐ None

140

Shape Set 11

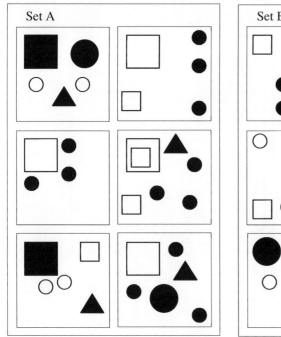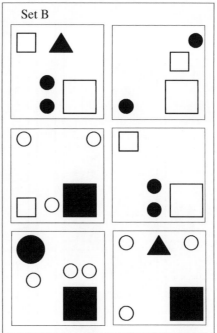

For each of the shapes below, decide whether they belong to Set A, Set B or Neither

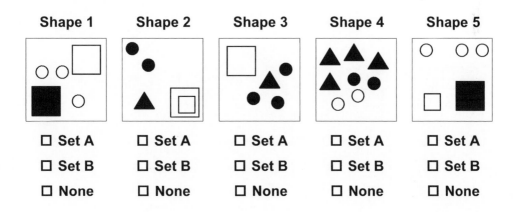

Shape 1	Shape 2	Shape 3	Shape 4	Shape 5
☐ Set A	☐ Set A	☐ Set A	☐ Set A	☐ Set A
☐ Set B	☐ Set B	☐ Set B	☐ Set B	☐ Set B
☐ None	☐ None	☐ None	☐ None	☐ None

Shape set 12

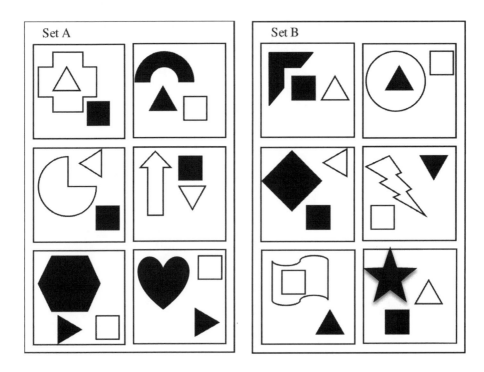

For each of the shapes below, decide whether they belong to Set A, Set B or Neither

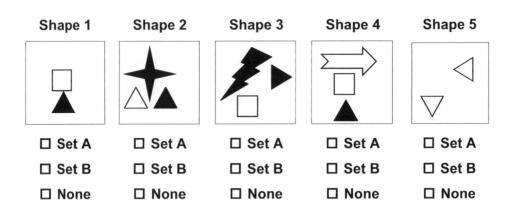

Shape 1	Shape 2	Shape 3	Shape 4	Shape 5
☐ Set A	☐ Set A	☐ Set A	☐ Set A	☐ Set A
☐ Set B	☐ Set B	☐ Set B	☐ Set B	☐ Set B
☐ None	☐ None	☐ None	☐ None	☐ None

Shape Set 13

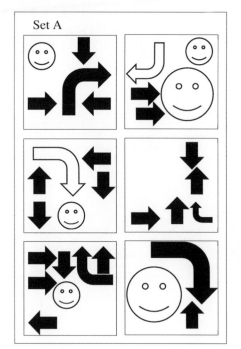

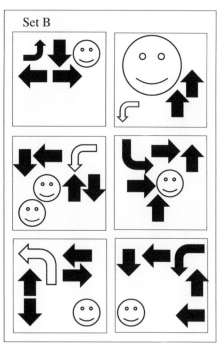

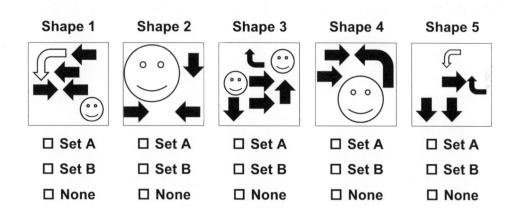

Shape 1	Shape 2	Shape 3	Shape 4	Shape 5
☐ Set A	☐ Set A	☐ Set A	☐ Set A	☐ Set A
☐ Set B	☐ Set B	☐ Set B	☐ Set B	☐ Set B
☐ None	☐ None	☐ None	☐ None	☐ None

143

Shape Set 14

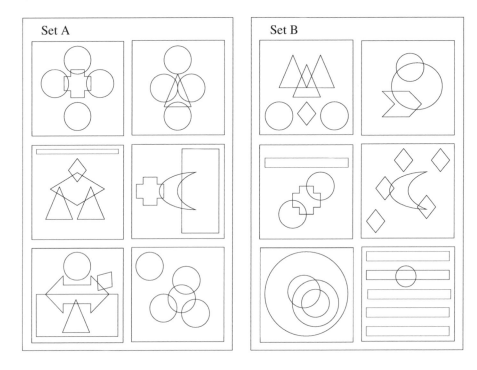

For each of the shapes below, decide whether they belong to Set A, Set B or neither:

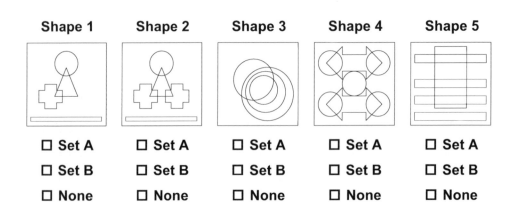

Shape 1	Shape 2	Shape 3	Shape 4	Shape 5
☐ Set A	☐ Set A	☐ Set A	☐ Set A	☐ Set A
☐ Set B	☐ Set B	☐ Set B	☐ Set B	☐ Set B
☐ None	☐ None	☐ None	☐ None	☐ None

Shape Set 15

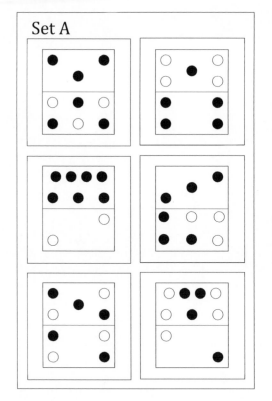

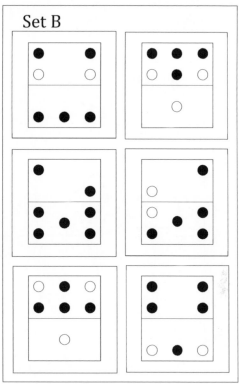

For each of the shapes below, decide whether they belong to Set A, Set B or neither

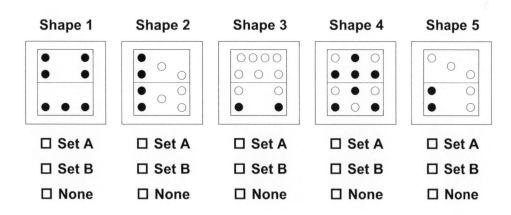

Shape 1	Shape 2	Shape 3	Shape 4	Shape 5
☐ Set A	☐ Set A	☐ Set A	☐ Set A	☐ Set A
☐ Set B	☐ Set B	☐ Set B	☐ Set B	☐ Set B
☐ None	☐ None	☐ None	☐ None	☐ None

Shape Set 16

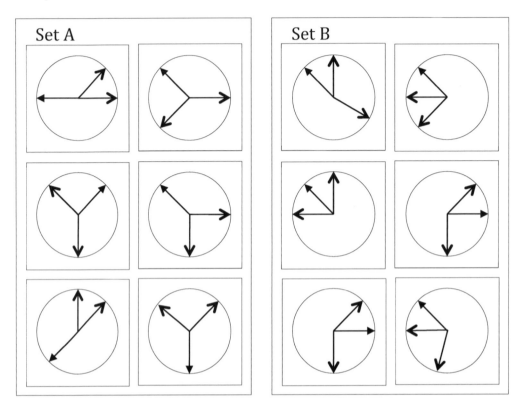

For each of the shapes below, decide whether they belong to Set A, Set B or neither

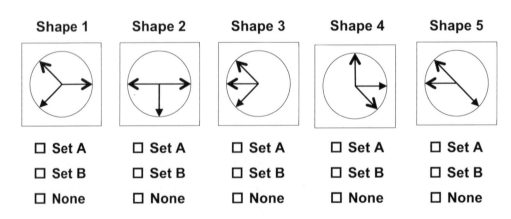

Shape 1	Shape 2	Shape 3	Shape 4	Shape 5
☐ Set A	☐ Set A	☐ Set A	☐ Set A	☐ Set A
☐ Set B	☐ Set B	☐ Set B	☐ Set B	☐ Set B
☐ None	☐ None	☐ None	☐ None	☐ None

146

Shape Set 17

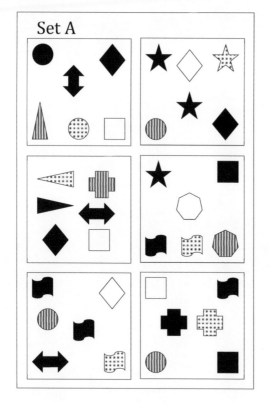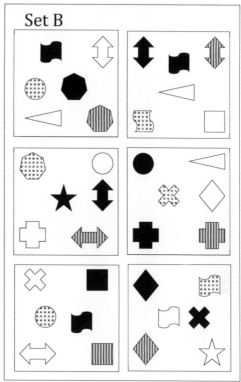

For each of the shapes below, decide whether they belong to Set A, Set B or neither

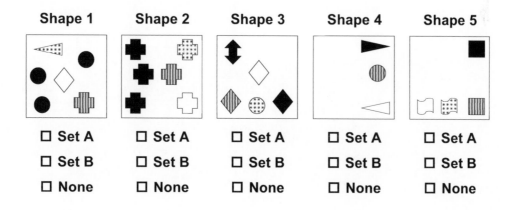

Shape 1	**Shape 2**	**Shape 3**	**Shape 4**	**Shape 5**
☐ Set A	☐ Set A	☐ Set A	☐ Set A	☐ Set A
☐ Set B	☐ Set B	☐ Set B	☐ Set B	☐ Set B
☐ None	☐ None	☐ None	☐ None	☐ None

Shape Set 18

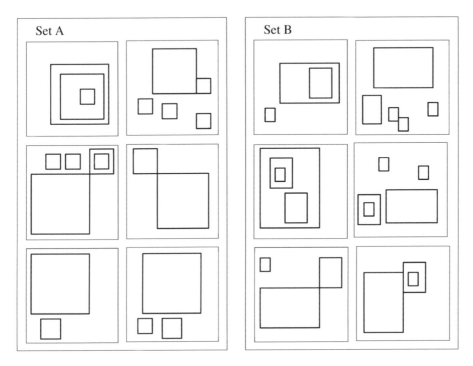

For each of the shapes below, decide whether they belong to Set A, Set B or neither

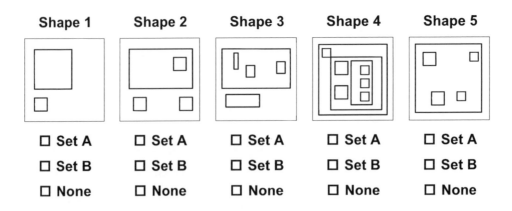

Shape 1	Shape 2	Shape 3	Shape 4	Shape 5
☐ Set A	☐ Set A	☐ Set A	☐ Set A	☐ Set A
☐ Set B	☐ Set B	☐ Set B	☐ Set B	☐ Set B
☐ None	☐ None	☐ None	☐ None	☐ None

Shape Set 19

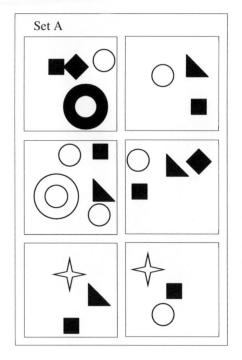
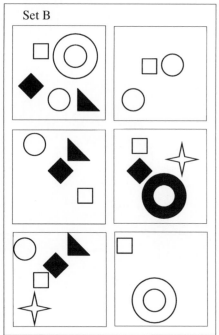

For each of the shapes below, decide whether they belong to Set A, Set B or neither

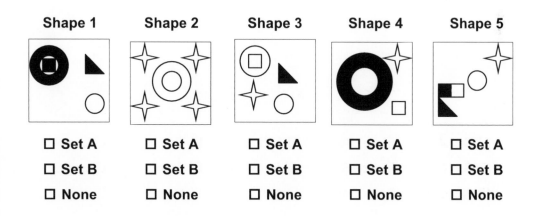

Shape 1	Shape 2	Shape 3	Shape 4	Shape 5
☐ Set A	☐ Set A	☐ Set A	☐ Set A	☐ Set A
☐ Set B	☐ Set B	☐ Set B	☐ Set B	☐ Set B
☐ None	☐ None	☐ None	☐ None	☐ None

Shape Set 20

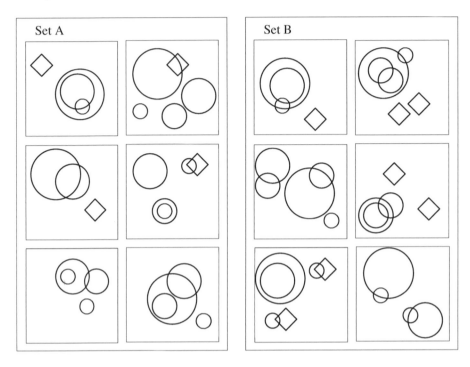

For each of the shapes below, decide whether they belong to Set A, Set B or neither

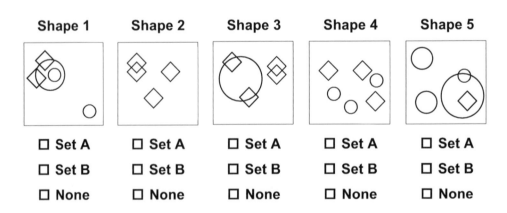

Shape 1	Shape 2	Shape 3	Shape 4	Shape 5
☐ Set A	☐ Set A	☐ Set A	☐ Set A	☐ Set A
☐ Set B	☐ Set B	☐ Set B	☐ Set B	☐ Set B
☐ None	☐ None	☐ None	☐ None	☐ None

Shape Set 21

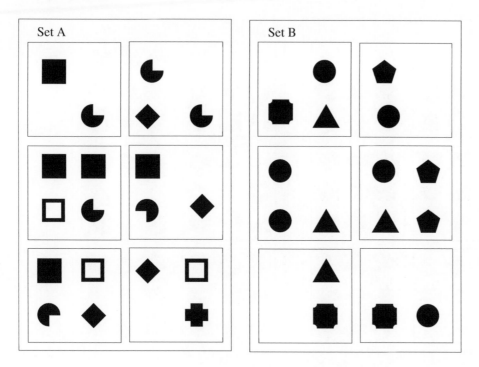

For each of the shapes below, decide whether they belong to Set A, Set B or neither

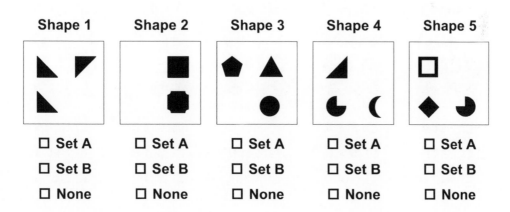

Shape 1	Shape 2	Shape 3	Shape 4	Shape 5
☐ Set A	☐ Set A	☐ Set A	☐ Set A	☐ Set A
☐ Set B	☐ Set B	☐ Set B	☐ Set B	☐ Set B
☐ None	☐ None	☐ None	☐ None	☐ None

Shape Set 22

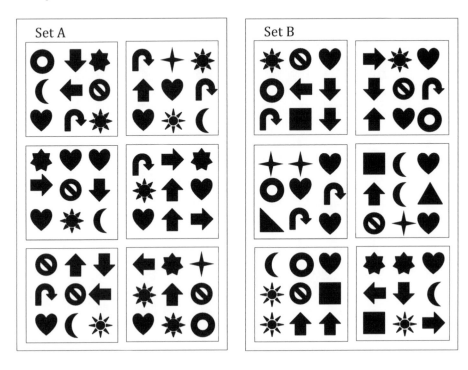

For each of the shapes below, decide whether they belong to Set A, Set B or neither

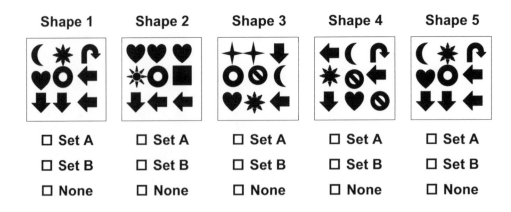

Shape 1	Shape 2	Shape 3	Shape 4	Shape 5
☐ Set A	☐ Set A	☐ Set A	☐ Set A	☐ Set A
☐ Set B	☐ Set B	☐ Set B	☐ Set B	☐ Set B
☐ None	☐ None	☐ None	☐ None	☐ None

Shape Set 23

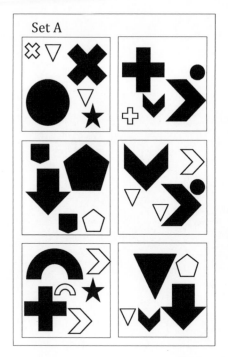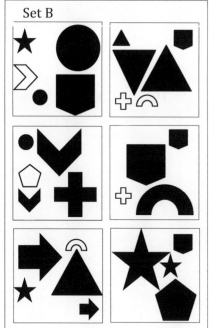

For each of the shapes below, decide whether they belong to Set A, Set B or neither

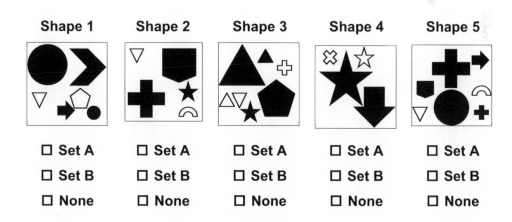

Shape 1	Shape 2	Shape 3	Shape 4	Shape 5
☐ Set A	☐ Set A	☐ Set A	☐ Set A	☐ Set A
☐ Set B	☐ Set B	☐ Set B	☐ Set B	☐ Set B
☐ None	☐ None	☐ None	☐ None	☐ None

Shape Set 24

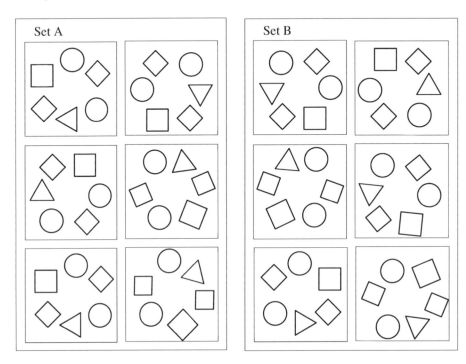

For each of the shapes below, decide whether they belong to Set A, Set B or neither

Shape 1	Shape 2	Shape 3	Shape 4	Shape 5
☐ Set A	☐ Set A	☐ Set A	☐ Set A	☐ Set A
☐ Set B	☐ Set B	☐ Set B	☐ Set B	☐ Set B
☐ None	☐ None	☐ None	☐ None	☐ None

154

Shape Set 25

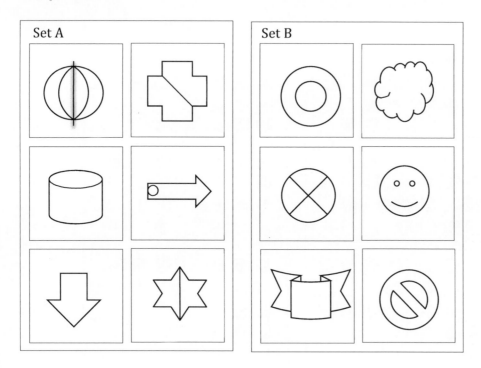

For each of the shapes below, decide whether they belong to Set A, Set B or neither

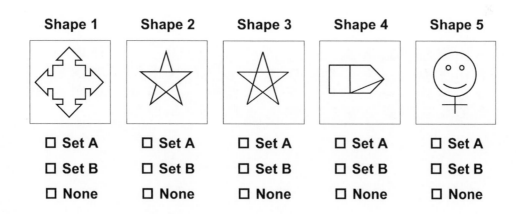

Shape 1	Shape 2	Shape 3	Shape 4	Shape 5
☐ Set A	☐ Set A	☐ Set A	☐ Set A	☐ Set A
☐ Set B	☐ Set B	☐ Set B	☐ Set B	☐ Set B
☐ None	☐ None	☐ None	☐ None	☐ None

Shape Set 26

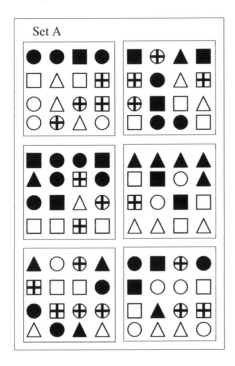
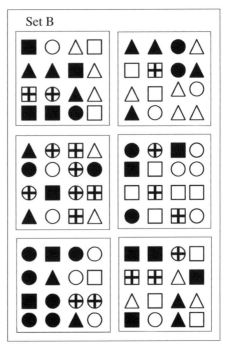

For each of the shapes below, decide whether they belong to Set A, Set B or neither

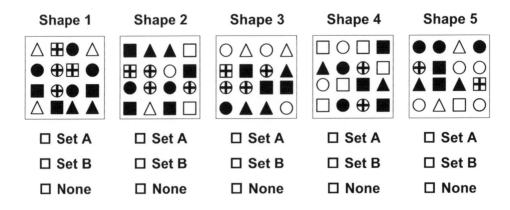

Shape 1	Shape 2	Shape 3	Shape 4	Shape 5
☐ Set A	☐ Set A	☐ Set A	☐ Set A	☐ Set A
☐ Set B	☐ Set B	☐ Set B	☐ Set B	☐ Set B
☐ None	☐ None	☐ None	☐ None	☐ None

156

Alternative Format Analytical Reasoning Questions:

1. Is A, B, C or D the next shape in the series?

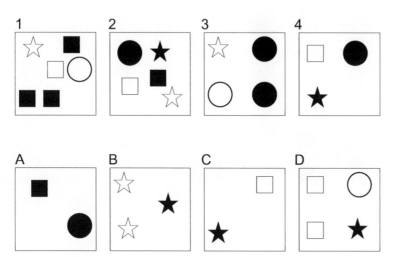

2. Is A, B, C or D the next shape in the series?

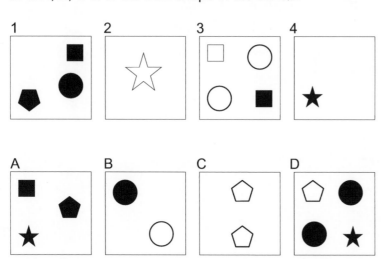

3. Is A, B, C or D the next shape in the series?

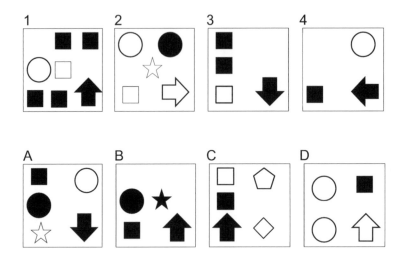

4. Is A, B, C or D the next shape in the series?

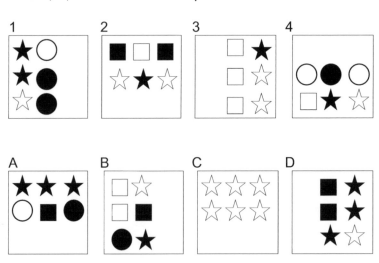

5.

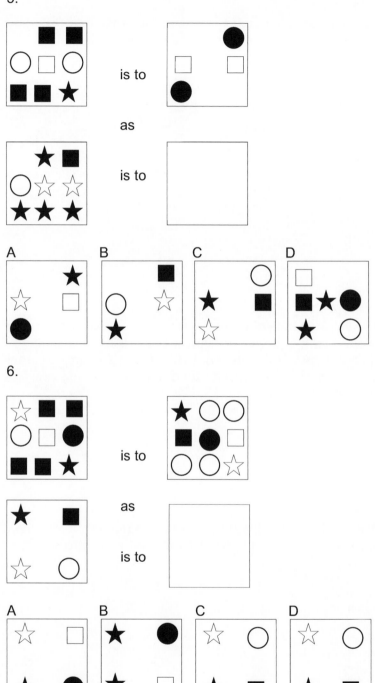

is to

as

is to

A   B   C   D

6.

is to

as

is to

A   B   C   D

Abstract Reasoning Practice Question Answers

Shape set 1: Set A contains an odd number of shapes, irrespective of shading. **Set B** contains an even number of shapes, none of which are shaded.

Shape 1: Set A
Shape 2: Neither
Shape 3: Set B
Shape 4: Neither
Shape 5: Set A

Shape set 2: All shapes in **set A** with four sides are shaded, whereas in **set B** all shapes without four sides are shaded.

Shape 1: Set B
Shape 2: Set B
Shape 3: Neither
Shape 4: Set A
Shape 5: Set A

Shape set 3: In **Set A** the presence of one or more circles means arrow up. If there is no circle present then the arrows are down. The presence of a triangle means arrows are shaded. In **Set B** the presence of one or more circles means arrows are down. If no circles are present then the arrows are up. The presence of a square means arrow shaded.

Shape 1: Set A
Shape 2: Neither
Shape 3: Set A
Shape 4: Neither
Shape 5: Set B

Shape set 4: In Set A the bottom left corner is blank and there are 2 curved edges per box. In Set B the top right corner is blank and there are 4 curved edges per box.

Shape 1: Set B
Shape 2: Neither
Shape 3: Neither
Shape 4: Neither
Shape 5: Neither

Shape set 5: In set A, the same shading is applied to two shapes diagonally opposite each other. The shapes in the other corners (also diagonally opposite

each other) are of the same type.
In set B, the shapes in the top and bottom right have the same shading. Shapes in the top left and bottom left are of the same type.

Shape 1: Set A
Shape 2: Set A
Shape 3: Neither
Shape 4: Set B
Shape 5: Neither

Shape set 6: In set A, if a black shape is counted as 2 and a white shape is counted as 1, the total is 9. In set B, if a black shape is counted as 2 and a white shape is counted as 1, the total is 7.

Shape 1: Set B
Shape 2: Neither
Shape 3: Set A
Shape 4: Set B
Shape 5: Neither

Shape set 7: In set A, there are 4 crossover points and two medium – sized objects. In set B there are 6 crossover points and one large object.

Shape 1: Neither
Shape 2: Set B
Shape 3: Neither
Shape 4: Set A
Shape 5: Set A

Shape set 8: In set A, the objects are all in the same rotational order. Shading is random. In set B, the shapes are shaded in the same rotational order but the shapes themselves are random.

Shape 1: Neither
Shape 2: Set A
Shape 3: Set B
Shape 4: Neither
Shape 5: Neither

Shape set 9: In set A, there is an even number of spots in the top box. If the number of spots in the top box is more than the number in the box below, the top spots are shaded. In set B, there are an odd number of spots in the top box. If the number of spots in the top box is more than the number below, the bottom box is shaded.

Shape 1: Set A
Shape 2: Set A
Shape 3: Set B
Shape 4: Set A
Shape 5: Set B

Shape set 10: In set A there are 10 shaded items, in rows of two and three alternately. In set B there are 10 non-shaded items in rows of two and three alternately.

Shape 1: Neither
Shape 2: Neither
Shape 3: Set A
Shape 4: Neither
Shape 5: Set A

Shape set 11: In set A, if there is a black box top left, there are two white circles. If there is a white box top left, there are three black circles. In set B, if there is a white box bottom right, there are two black circles. If there is a black box bottom right, there are three white circles. All other shapes are distractors.

Shape 1: Neither
Shape 2: Set B
Shape 3: Set A
Shape 4: Neither
Shape 5: Set B

Shape set 12: Both sets contain a large object in the top left hand corner. In set A, if the large object is white, the box also contains a black square and a white triangle. If the large object is black, the box also contains a black triangle and a white box.

In set B, the reverse is true. If the large object is black, there is also a white triangle and a black square. If the large object is white, there is a white square and black triangle.

Shape 1: Neither
Shape 2: Neither
Shape 3: Set A
Shape 4: Set B
Shape 5: Neither

Shape set 13: In set A there is a curved arrow going clockwise in each box. In set B, there is a curved arrow going anti-clockwise in each box.

Shape 1: Set B
Shape 2: Neither
Shape 3: Set A
Shape 4: Set B
Shape 5: Neither

Shape set 14: Set A contains shapes that intersect at 6 points. Set B contains shapes that intersect at 4 points.

Shape 1: Set B
Shape 2: Set A
Shape 3: Set A
Shape 4: Neither
Shape 5: Neither

Shape set 15: In Set A, the total number of spots is 9. There is an even number of spots in the lower half. In Set B, the total number of spots is 7. There are an odd number of spots in the lower half. The shading in both sets is irrelevant.

Shape 1: Set B
Shape 2: Neither
Shape 3: Neither
Shape 4: Neither
Shape 5: Neither

Shape set 16: In Set A, there is 135 degrees between the smaller arrow and one of the larger ones. The other large arrow points randomly. In Set B, there is 45 degrees between the smaller arrow and one of the larger ones. The other arrow points randomly.

Shape 1: Set A
Shape 2: Neither
Shape 3: Set B
Shape 4: Set B
Shape 5: Set A

Shape set 17: Set A contains 3 black shapes, 1 dotted shape the same as one of the black shapes, 1 striped shape and 1 white shape. Set B contains 2 black shapes, 1 striped shape the same as one of the black shapes, 1 dotted shape and 2 white shapes.

Shape 1: Neither
Shape 2: Set A
Shape 3: Neither
Shape 4: Neither
Shape 5: Neither

Shape set 18: In set A, all the shapes are made from squares, in set B all the shapes are rectangles.

Shape 1: Set A
Shape 2: Neither
Shape 3: Set B
Shape 4: Neither
Shape 5: Set A

Shape set 19: Set A contains a black square in each box. Set B contains a white square in each box.

Shape 1: Set A
Shape 2: Neither
Shape 3: Set B
Shape 4: Set B
Shape 5: Neither

Shape set 20: In set A, there are two points where lines cross each other. In set B, there are 4 points where lines cross each other.

Shape 1: Set B
Shape 2: Set A
Shape 3: Neither
Shape 4: Neither
Shape 5: Set A

Shape set 21: All shapes in set A have at least one right angle. None of the shapes in set B have a right angle.
Shape 1: Set A
Shape 2: Neither
Shape 3: Set B
Shape 4: Neither
Shape 5: Set A

Shape set 22: In set A, there is a heart in the bottom left corner of each box. In set B, there is a heart in the top right corner of each box.

Shape 1: Neither
Shape 2: Set B
Shape 3: Set A
Shape 4: Neither
Shape 5: Neither

Shape set 23: There are two large black objects in all of the boxes. In set A, there is a smaller version of one of them in white. In set B, there is a smaller version of one of them in black.

Shape 1: Set B
Shape 2: Neither
Shape 3: Set B
Shape 4: Set A
Shape 5: Set B

Shape set 24: In set A all the shapes are the same and in the same order but are rotated. Set B is the mirror image of set B and the boxes are also rotated.

Shape 1: Set B
Shape 2: Set A
Shape 3: Neither
Shape 4: Neither
Shape 5: Set B

Shape set 25: In set A, all the images can be drawn without taking a pencil off the paper and without going over a line twice. In set B, to draw the images the pencil must be taken off the paper or a line must be drawn twice.

Shape 1: Set A
Shape 2: Set B
Shape 3: Set A
Shape 4: Set A
Shape 5: Set B

Shape set 26: In set A there are four identical shapes in each corner. The top two are shaded and the bottom two aren't. In set B there are four identical shapes in each corner. The left two are shaded, the right two aren't.

Shape 1: Neither
Shape 2: Set B
Shape 3: Neither
Shape 4: Neither
Shape 5: Set A

Alternative Format Analytical Reasoning Answers

1. **C**. There are a decreasing number of shapes in each set. The types of shape are distractors but the shading is reduced alternately (i.e. one less white one then one less black one and so on).

2. **C**. The total number of sides in each set is 10. Number, shading and type of shapes are distractors.

3. **B**. The arrow in the bottom right corner is rotating clockwise. There is also always a square in the bottom left corner.

4. **B**. The area with no shapes is rotating clockwise. Type and shading of the shapes are distractors.

5. **A**. The bottom left shape has swapped positions with the one above it. The top right shape has swapped with the one below it. All swapped shapes have the taken on their opposite shading. The other shapes have all disappeared.

6. **C**. Stars have changed shading. Circles have become squares and changed shading. Squares have become circles and have changed shading.

Chapter 4

Decision Analysis

Decision analysis

UKCAT says: 'The test assesses the ability to make decisions in situations of uncertainty. It requires candidates to make informed judgements with information that is incomplete, complex and ambiguous. Using a deciphering scenario, the test requires a move from logical reasoning to decisions requiring increasing degrees of judgement'.

You have 32 minutes to read the instructions and answer 28 items. Allowing 1 minute to read the instructions, this gives you **an average of 66 seconds to answer each item.**

The test requires you to find the best interpretation of a coded message. You are given a key to the code, which will be expanded over the course of the 26 questions. The coded information will at times be incomplete or odd, but there will always be a 'best' answer and you must use your judgement to decide which it is.

You will be given a brief scenario to set the scene and then a table of codes. Initially this will be simple and contain 'operator words' and 'specific info'. An operator word would be something like 'reduce' or 'increase'. Specific info would be code words relating to the scenario. After approximately 10 questions the code will be expanded to include further 'complex info' (more scenario-related words) and 'reaction/outcome' codes, such as 'happy' or 'finished'. Most of the questions involve the 'best interpretation' of a code. There will be a few (usually 4-6) towards the end of the test that either requires you to give the most helpful additional code word or the best way to code a message (see examples).

Why is Decision Analysis in the exam?

This part of the exam looks at how you organise information and make judgements and interpretations about it. Sometimes parts of the information will be incomplete and you must use your judgement to make the most sensible and accurate interpretation. This is a skill you will require throughout your career, whether it is communicating with colleagues, taking histories from patients or interpreting written information in journals or newspapers.

Top tips:

- First, translate the code literally and write it down.
- Some words are used to modify others and these may be 'linked' to other bits of code, for example by being in brackets or not separated by a comma. Make sure you keep this 'linking' in your answer if you can

- Try not to have any extra information in your answer if you can help it - keep it as simple as you can
- Try and stick to the order the code is given in if possible
- Consider the different meanings of words, for example 'light' can be interpreted as 'not heavy' or 'sunlight'
- Look out for small changes such as tenses or plurals
- Questions tend to get harder and longer towards the end of the test
- There are 2 different types of question towards the end of the set of 26 - you may be asked to identify the best extra code word(s) to complete a coded message or to identify the beset code to convey a certain message.

Worked Examples

Spy Codes

A spy gives and receives messages via text. To make them difficult to interpret he uses a code previously agreed with his spymaster. Whilst working for the ministry of intelligence, you intercept some of his messages. Your agency has developed a basic interpretation sheet:

Operators		Specific Information	
A	More	1	Personal
B	Generalise	2	Missile
C	Future	3	Aircraft
D	Opposite	4	Danger
E	Combine	5	People
F	Many	6	Help
G	Release		

1. What is the best interpretation of the following code?

1, C, (D, 4)

I stake my future against danger
Safety is my priority
I am safe
I will be safe
My future is dangerous

Literal translation: Personal, Future (Opposite, Danger)

Personal can be interpreted as 'I' or 'My'
Future can mean 'the future', or give a future tense
'Opposite' and 'Danger' are linked by brackets, indicating they should be interpreted together. The opposite of 'danger' is 'safety'.
Putting it all together, **'I will be safe'** is the simplest direct translation that does not add any meaning and uses all the code.

2. What is the best interpretation of the following code?

E (F (2, 3, 5)), (D, 6)

The air force has been a nuisance lately
There has not been much help at the airport
Many people have complained about the airport
The air force was unable to help to start with
Most help did not come from the RAF

Literal translation: Combine (Many (Missile, Aircraft, People)), (Opposite, Help)

At first glance, none of the answers seem to fit. There is additional meaning in all of the answers so you have to use your judgement to decide which is best.

Combine (Many (Missile, Aircraft, People)) can be interpreted as 'the air force' or 'the RAF'. 'Airport' is a possible translation but not so good as most airports do not contain missiles.
'(Opposite, Help)' can be interpreted as 'a nuisance' and it is difficult to find another good interpretation of it in the other answers.
Therefore, even though 'lately' has not been coded for, the correct answer is 'The air force has been a nuisance lately'

Your intelligence agency then manages to translate more of the code:

Operators		Specific Information		Complex Information		Reactions / Outcomes	
A	More	1	Personal	100	Fast	P	Fear
B	Generalise	2	Missile	200	Hold	Q	Trust
C	Future	3	Aircraft	300	Alive	R	Surprise
D	Opposite	4	Danger	400	General	S	Worried
E	Combine	5	People	500	Think	T	Hope
F	Many	6	Help				
G	Release						

170

3. What is the best interpretation of the following code?

400, S, (A, F), 5, (D, 300)

Most dead people are generally worried
The General is worried about all the people that have been killed
Dead people all worry the General
All the people are worried about killing the General
General worry kills most people

Literal translation: General, Worried, (More, Many), People, (Opposite, Alive)

In this example, 'more' and 'many' need to be combined. You could interpret this as 'more than many' which could be 'all' or 'most'. 'Opposite' and 'alive' can be combined to give something to do with death, such as 'dead' or 'killed'. All of the translations contain only the code given and use all of it. The answer that makes the most sense and users the code in the correct order is 'The General is worried about all the people that have been killed'.

4. You hope to send a fake message back to the spy. What is the best way to code the following message?

A few people would like to kill the General

400, (D, 300), 5
(D, F), 5, (D, 6) 400
(D, F), 5, T, (D, 300), 400
400, (D, F), 5, (D, 300), T
400, (D, 300), T

(D, F), 5, T, (D, 300), 400 translates as (Opposite, Many), People, Hope (Opposite, Alive), General
The opposite of 'many' could be 'few' and 'hope' could be translated as 'would like to' and this code gives an accurate message in a sensible order so is the correct answer.

General, (Opposite, Alive), People This does not contain enough information to transmit the message. There is more code available that would help.

(D, F), 5, (D, 6) 400 translates as (Opposite, Many), People, (Opposite, Help) General. It's difficult to understand why 'Opposite, Help' could be interpreted as meaning 'Would like to'

400, (D, F), 5, (D, 300), T translates as General, (Opposite, Alive), People, (Opposite, Many), Hope
Although this contains all the code required to give the message, they are not in the correct order and so this is not the best answer.

400, (D, 300), T translates as General, (Opposite Many), Hope. This clearly does not contain enough information.

Top tip: Before translating all the codes, think what parts of the code you would use to write the message and write them down. You may well find a very similar answer.

5. You wish to send the following message:

Most of the population believe the army will lose to the air force

Which two words would be the most useful additions to the code to help you send this message?

Troops
Majority
Defeat
Inhabitants
Conclude

Think about which part of the code is already available. In this case, 'Most' could be coded for with (More, Many). 'Population' could be coded for with (Many, People). Believe could be 'Think'.

It is most difficult to code for 'Lose' and 'Army'. Therefore the two words that are most useful would be 'Troops' and 'Defeat'

Decision Analysis Exercise

Take 1 minute to read these instructions.

You will be asked to solve a code and make the best interpretation of its meaning. As you progress through the questions, the code will become more complex. The last few questions of the exam will involve identifying extra code that is required to complete a coded message and identifying the best way to code a message.

You have 10 minutes to answer 8 questions. Try and answer all the questions. There is no negative marking.

Some astronauts and their controllers on Earth develop a code to communicate with each other. Interpret the following messages as best you can.

Operators		Specific Information	
A	Develop	1	People
B	Down	2	Us
C	Negative	3	Building
D	Shrink	4	Earth
E	Ignite	5	Moon
F	Collapse	6	Stars
G	Add	7	Country
H	Apply	8	Sky
I	Overlay	9	Air
J	Distribute	10	Hot
K	Separate	11	Frozen
L	Evolve	12	Electricity
M	Greater	13	Fuel
		14	Water
		15	Ice

1. What is the best interpretation of the following code?

(1, 5, 6), B, 14

The people in space are running out of water
The astronauts landed in the ocean
It rained on the astronauts
There is not much water in space
The aliens have run out of water

173

2. What is the best interpretation of the following code?

G (8,6,5), A, 11, 14

Ice forms at night-time
Ice is present on the moon and some stars
It's snowing from the heavens
There is ice in space
It is very cold in space

3. What is the best interpretation of the following code?

C, E, 13, H, (K, 2, 8), B

Burning the fuel is what keeps us in the sky.
Don't ignite the fuel or we'll be blown out of the sky.
If the engine goes out we'll fall out of the sky.
Separate us from the fuel whilst we're in the air.
When the fuel runs out we'll start our descent.

4. What is the best interpretation of the following code?

(110,1), (M, 101), (110, 4)

It took a long time before people evolved on earth
People evolved after the formation of earth
People evolved on earth
People have not been around since time began
There are more people on earth than any other planet

5. What is the best interpretation of the following code?

114(D), (101, 102), H, K (2,6)

The distance between us and the stars is increasing
The universe is contracting
The universe is expanding
The universe will shrink as time increases
We are separated from the stars by time and space

6. What is the best interpretation of the following code?

105, 4, 109, (5, 6), (114, 5, 6)

The moon and the stars rotate around the earth.
A spinning planet created the moon and stars
Night and day were created by the turning of the Earth
Daylight begins when the Earth rotates from night time
The turning of the Earth causes night and day

7. Which two code words would be most useful to send the following message?

There will not be much fuel to start the faulty motor

Engine
Future
Plenty
Broken
Soon

8. What is the best way to code the following message?

Ice covers the whole of the moon

15, I, 5
(114, 208), 15, 5
15, 5, I, (114, 208)
5, (15, I, (114, 208))
15, H, 5, (114, D)

Answers:

1. (1, 5, 6), B, 14 translates as **(People, Moon, Stars), Down, Water**

The correct answer is 'The astronauts landed in the ocean'

(People, Moon, Stars) are all linked to form 'astronauts'. 'Down' and 'water' are then used to give 'landed in the ocean'. The code is used in the correct order and an appropriate interpretation of all the code has been made.

'The people in space are running out of water' is close but does not link 'people, moon, stars,' in to one meaning. This option would have been a strong contender had the brackets not been present
'It rained on the astronauts' is a possibility but changes the order of the code and so is not as good as the correct answer
'There is not much water in space' does not use 'people'
'The aliens have run out of water' switches 'people' to 'aliens'

2. G (8,6,5), A, 11, 14 translates to **Add (Sky, Stars, Moon), Develop, Frozen, Water**

The correct answer is **'Ice forms at night-time'**

Add (Sky, Stars, Moon) can be interpreted as 'night-time'
'Frozen water' is 'Ice'
'Develop' is 'Forms'

'Ice is present on the moon and some stars' is not correct because the correct answer offers a better interpretation of 'develop' and there is no use of 'sky'

'It's snowing from the heavens' is a possible correct answer, but is not as good an interpretation as the correct answer as there is no use of 'develop'

'There is ice in space' does not use 'develop'

'It is very cold in space' does not use 'water'

3. C, E, 13, H, K (2, 8), B translates as **Negative Ignite Fuel, Apply, (Separate, Us, Sky), Down**

If the engine goes out we'll fall out of the sky is the correct answer

176

'Apply' can be interpreted as linking the other parts of the code.

'Negative ignite fuel' can be interpreted as the fuel is not lighting - i.e. the engine is not on.

'Separate (Us, Sky), Down' can be interpreted as we will be separate from the sky by going down i.e. we'll fall out of the sky

'Burning the fuel is what keeps us in the sky' is incorrect because there is no use of 'negative'

'Don't ignite the fuel or we'll be blown out of the sky' is close but requires the use of extra coding to describe being 'blown' out of the sky

'Separate us from the fuel whilst we're in the air' is wrong because 'Separate' should be linked to 'Us, Sky' rather than fuel. There is also no use of 'down'

'When the fuel runs out we'll start our descent' is not such a good translation because 'negative ignite fuel' is better interpreted as 'when the engine goes out' rather than 'when the fuel runs out'

4. (110,1), (M, 101), (110, 4) translates as **Start (People), Greater (Time), Start (Earth)**

'People evolved after the formation of earth' is the correct answer. It links the 'start' of 'people' (evolution of people) to the 'start' of the 'earth' (formation of earth). The 'Greater, Time' part of the code can be interpreted as 'people' or 'earth' have been around longer - and in this answer it is implied that the earth has been around for longer

'It took a long time before people evolved on earth' does not link 'Earth' specifically with 'Time' as implied by the code

'People evolved on earth'. Although 'Start' can be interpreted as 'Evolve' there is no linking of 'Start' to Earth in this answer

'People have not been around since time began'. 'Greater' has not been used

'There are more people on earth than any other planet'. This answer includes references to other planets that are not in the code

5. (114, D), (101, 102), H, K (2,6) translates as **Opposite (Shrink), (Time, Space), Apply, Separate (Us, Stars)**.

'The universe is expanding' is the correct answer. An increase (Opposite (Shrink), in time and space (the fabric of the universe) which is then applied to the separation between us and the stars may be interpreted as the universe is expanding.

'The distance between us and the stars is increasing' does not interpret expansion of 'time'

'The universe is contracting' does not make use of 'opposite'

'The universe will shrink as time increases' does not make use of 'opposite'

'We are separated from the stars by time and space' does not make use of 'opposite (shrink)'

6. 105, 4, 109, (5, 6), (114, 5, 6) translates as **'Revolve, Earth, Create, (Moon, Stars), (Opposite, Moon, Stars)**

The turning of the Earth causes night and day is the correct answer. ('Moon, Stars) can be linked to give 'night', the opposite of which is 'day'.

'The moon and the stars rotate around the earth' does not use all the code and is in the wrong order.

'A spinning planet created the moon and stars' does not use all the code and 'Earth' is mentioned specifically, rather than 'a planet'.

'Night and day were created by the turning of the Earth' is a possibility but the order is not as good as in the original answer.

'Daylight begins when the Earth rotates from night time' is another possibility but changes the order of the code.

7. The most useful code words would be **'Engine'** and **'Future'**

'Sparse' and 'Fuel' and 'Start' are available in the code and can be used to give 'not much fuel to start'.

'Break' could be used for 'faulty'

The options we are then left with are 'Engine', 'Future' and 'Soon'. 'Engine' is clearly useful for giving 'motor'.

We are then left with trying to convey 'There will (not) be'. 'Future' is better than 'soon' as it does not imply a timescale, only a tense.

8. 15, I, 5 is translated as Ice, Overlay, Moon. This is nice and simple and in the right order, but there is no sense of 'the whole' of the moon.

(114, 208), 15, 5 translates as (Opposite, Sparse), Ice, Moon and could be interpreted as 'There is lots of ice on the moon'

15, 5, I, (114, 208) translates as Ice, Moon, Overlay, (Opposite, Sparse) and contains all of the words to give the required message, but in the wrong order.

5, (15, I, (114, 208)) Moon, (Ice, Overlay, (Opposite, Sparse) is the correct answer as it contains all the words to give the message. Although they are not in the correct order, 'Opposite, Sparse' is linked to 'Ice' and 'Overlay' and so gives the best attempt ago conveying the message.

15, H, 5, (114, D) translates as 'Ice, Apply, Moon, (Opposite, Shrink)' and this implies ice is covering a 'growing' moon. It does not come close to conveying the correct message.

Decision Analysis Practice Questions

Depending on how many code questions you do, allow yourself the following time:

1 code: 66 seconds
2 codes: 1 minute and 12 seconds
5 codes: 5 minutes and 30 seconds
10 codes: 11 minutes
20 codes: 22 minutes
28 codes: 31 minutes

Code Set 1

Operators		Specific Info	
A	Sleep	1	Air
B	Above	2	Gravity
C	Underneath	3	Weight
D	Time	4	Rope
E	Forward	5	Tough
F	Opposite	6	Loose
G	Against	7	Bricks
H	Toward	8	Helium
I	Until	9	Lead
J	Again	10	Wheel
K	Stop	11	Small
L	Expect	12	Thirsty
M	Contains	13	Blind
N	More	14	Animals
O	Most	15	Planet
P	Not	16	Solar System
		17	Washed

What is the best interpretation of the following coded messages?

180

Code 1:

2, M (15,16)

a) Gravitational forces between planets in the solar system are negligible.
b) Gravitational forces work in opposite directions between the planets in the solar system.
c) Gravity brings celestial bodies together.
d) Gravity acts on the planet in our solar system.
e) Gravity keeps the planet in the solar system

Code 2:

E 10, (K, P) (I, G, 4)

a) Roll the wheel forward until the slack is taken up by the rope.
b) Start moving the wheel forward with the rope.
c) Stop the wheel from moving by using the rope.
d) The wheel is pulled forward by the rope.
e) The wheels are stopped from moving by the rope.

Code 3:

L (11, 1), 15 (11, 2)

a) A planet with a lack of gravity leads to a lack of air.
b) Don't expect to be able to breathe on a planet with low gravity.
c) Expect planets without air to have no gravity.
d) Planets without air have no gravity.
e) This planet does not have enough air or gravity.

Code 4:

(N, 2, 15), (L, N, 3)

a) Expect things to be heavier on a planet with higher gravity.
b) Gravity causes things to become heavy
c) Gravity is dependent upon the size of the planet
d) Most planets have more gravity than this
e) The bigger the planet the greater the effect of gravity

Code 5:

(F, K), (6,7), (C, 3)

a) Bricks are becoming loose under the weight.
b) The loose bricks underneath can support the weight.
c) The weight is held underneath the loose bricks.
d) There are no loose supporting bricks.
e) Underneath the weight are loose bricks.

Code 6:

(F, O) 14, (H, K), (E, D, 11)

a) Some species have been around a short time
b) It only takes a short time for a species to become extinct.
c) Most of the animals will make the crossing in a very short time.
d) A few animals will become extinct soon
e) Without stopping some of the animals will not arrive in time.

Code 7:

F (O 11), 14 (O 5)

a) The least tough animals are smallest
b) Tough animals are bigger
c) The toughest animal is the largest
d) The largest animals are toughest
e) Large beasts are tough

Code 8:

(E 1), 14, (H 12)

a) Windy animals become thirsty
b) There is dry air in front of the animals
c) The air moves forward towards the thirsty animals
d) Dry wind makes the animals thirsty
e) The animals are becoming thirsty in the wind

Code 9:

(9 3), 17 (F H)

a) The heavy weights have been washed
b) The anchor has been washed away
c) The heavy lead weight has been washed
d) Don't clean the metal weights
e) The lead weight is dirty

Now also use the extra code on the following page.

Code 10:

103 (8, 201, G2)

a) A helium balloon will rise.
b) A true helium balloon is unaffected by gravity.
c) Anti-gravity can be compared to a helium balloon.
d) Helium balloons don't feel gravity.
e) True anti-gravity is no different to a helium balloon.

Code 11:

203, (202, F, 105), (N, F, 204), 109 (D, 108)

a) I have been stung many times this year.
b) Make the bees produce sweeter honey this time.
c) The bees are more aggressive than they were.
d) The bees have produced very little honey this time.
e) The honey is even sweeter this year.

Code 12:

(211, 106), 210 (105 205), (H, 101)

a) Pain and suffering are less.
b) Suffering is caused by the inability to relieve pain.
c) There is no suffering without pain.
d) To understand suffering we must understand pain.
e) Understanding the pathways of pain will help us to reduce suffering

Operators		Specific Info	
A	Sleep	1	Air
B	Above	2	Gravity
C	Underneath	3	Weight
D	Time	4	Rope
E	Forward	5	Tough
F	Opposite	6	Loose
G	Against	7	Bricks
H	Toward	8	Helium
I	Until	9	Lead
J	Again	10	Wheel
K	Stop	11	Small
L	Expect	12	Thirsty
M	Contains	13	Blind
N	More	14	Animals
O	Most	15	Planet
P	Not	16	Solar System
		17	Washed

Complex Info		Extra info	
101	Explain	201	Balloon
102	Suspend	202	Bees
103	True	203	Liquid
104	Attack	204	Sour
105	Disassemble	205	Pain
106	Less	206	Magic
107	Apart	207	Unknown
108	Back	208	Life
109	Compared	209	Personal
110	Attach	210	Method
111	Allow		
112	Suspect		
113	Generalise		

184

Code 13:

209, 113, G (K, 208), 210 (102, 4)

a) I am against the death penalty.
b) I believe hanging is a cruel way to die.
c) I believe most people are against hanging.
d) I do not wish to be hung.
e) I tried to commit suicide.

Code 14:

(N, 3), (9, 109, 8), (112, N, 2)

a) Gravity exerts a greater force on lead than helium.
b) I suspect lead is heavier than helium.
c) Lead is heavier than helium but I suspect both are equally affected by gravity.
d) Lead is heavier than helium, probably because it is more affected by gravity.
e) Lead is more likely to fall due to gravity.

Code 15:

209, 112, 207, 15, 208, 111

a) My suspicion is that many undiscovered planets support life
b) I think a planet not yet discovered will support life
c) I am unsure whether other planets allow life
d) My belief is to allow unknown life to continue on the planet
e) It is unknown whether there is another planet that supports life

Code 16:

209, 111, N (209, 208)

a) Allow me more of a home life
b) I allow life to be more personal
c) My life is more than I expected
d) Balancing personal and work lives is difficult
e) Many personal lives are allowed

Code 17:

9, 104, (F, 105), 7, 208

a) I led the attack on the people in the building
b) Lead the attack on DNA
c) Lead is responsible for many attacks on the building blocks of life
d) Build a life and lead it well
e) Lead can destroy the building blocks of life

Code 18:

113, (208, M, 205) (204, 208)
a) Life usually contains pain which makes people unhappy
b) Generally, if life contains pain people are unhappy
c) A life full of pain is an unhappy life
d) Usually, lives containing pain are unhappy lives
e) Pain in life leads to bitterness

Code 19:

(N, 12) 14, (F, 208), (106, D)

a) A very thirsty animal dies quickly
b) Dehydrated animals die quickly
c) It takes less time for a dehydrated animal to die
d) The thirstiest animals deteriorate in less time
e) The more thirsty and animal is, the less time it takes to die

Code 20:

(202, 203), 209, 110 (A, 106)

a) My bees are unable to sleep
b) I blame my insomnia on my bees
c) Honey helps me sleep
d) Honey, I can't sleep
e) I'm sleepless in honey

Code 21:

Which would be the most useful additional code to convey the following?

I can see the nuts on the wheel are tight

a) Nut
b) Secure
c) Wheel
d) Me
e) Visualise

Code 22:

Which would be the two most useful additional codes to convey the following?

Without looking, tell me the correct number

a) Advise, Accurate
b) Accurate, Sum
c) Discuss, Outside
d) Advise, Quantity
e) Excluding, See

Code 23:

Which would be the two most useful additional codes to convey the following?

Take the animals up to the mountain pasture

a) Bring, Meadow
b) High, Meadow
c) Fauna, High
d) Alpine, Fauna
e) Herds, Fauna

Code 24:

Choose the best code for the following sentence:

The heaviest wheels are not durable

a) L, 5, F, 3, J
b) 3, 10, 5
c) (O, 3), 10, P
d) (O 3), (J 10), P, 5
e) (N 3), (N 10), 5

Code 25:

Choose the best code for the following sentence:

Tie the loose animals up

a) 14, G, H, 6
b) 4, 6, 14, (H B)
c) (F C), 14, 4
d) 4, 6, 14, G
e) 6, 14, M 4, (F C)

Code 26:

Choose the best code for the following sentence:

I expect there is more unknown life

a) 209, L, N, (208 207)
b) 207, 208, M, 15
c) 209, (208 207), L, N
d) O, (207 208) L, 209
e) 14, 207, 15

Code Set 2

Operators		Specific Info	
200	Before	A	Woman
201	Possibility	B	Prepared
202	Opposite	C	Personal
203	Plural	D	Heavy
204	Without	E	Soldier
205	Enlarge	F	Hill
206	Combine	G	Forest
207	Seldom	H	Food
208	Reduce	I	Child
209	Common	J	Spanish
210	Copy	K	Liquid
		L	Man
		M	Love

Code 1:

A, M, (203, I)

a) The woman loves children
b) The child is loved by the woman
c) Women love children
d) The woman loves the child
e) Children love the woman

Code 2:

J, (208, M), H

a) I love eating Spanish food
b) Everyone likes Spanish food
c) Spaniards love food
d) The Spanish like food
e) Spanish food is excellent

Code 3:

206 (L, A, I), 205

a) Many families are getting bigger
b) The family is very fat
c) The family is getting bigger
d) The people are huge
e) The family is growing rapidly

Code 4:

C, (B, 202), (H, 204)

a) I am ready for hunger
b) I was not ready for the famine
c) Without food I can never be ready
d) I am not ready unless I am hungry
e) I am ready to eat

Code 5:

(203, C), (204, K)

a) I cannot be without lots of fluid
b) I cannot be without fluid
c) We are thirsty
d) We need more water
e) We are very thirsty

Code 6:

203 (202, I), M, G

a) Many children love the forest
b) Forests are loved by the elderly
c) Lots of children are scared of the forest
d) The elderly love the woodland
e) Old people don't like the wood

Code 7:

(205, E), (200, M), H

a) The obese soldier loves food
b) The fat soldier loved food
c) The soldiers love food
d) Many soldiers loved eating
e) A larger soldier puts food before love

Code 8:

206 (L, A), 209, (204, K)

a) Many, many couples are thirsty
b) Often couples need more liquid
c) Many couples are without water
d) Without water, many people will die
e) Men and women are often without water

Code 9:

(205, C), 206 (H, K), 201, D

a) These provisions may make me very fat
b) The heaviness of the supplies could make things difficult
c) Our food and water might weigh too much
d) My provisions could be heavy
e) Our supplies may be heavy

Code 10:

206 (L, A, I), 209, (204, H)

a) Without food the family may starve
b) Husband and wife usually are without food
c) Men, women and children commonly go without food
d) The family is often hungry
e) Being often without food brings people together

Operators		Specific Info	
200	Before	A	Woman
201	Possibility	B	Prepared
202	Opposite	C	Personal
203	Plural	D	Heavy
204	Without	E	Soldier
205	Enlarge	F	Hill
206	Combine	G	Forest
207	Seldom	H	Food
208	Reduce	I	Child
209	Common	J	Spanish
210	Copy	K	Liquid
		L	Man
		M	Love

Complex Info		Extra info	
!	Fierce	10	Horse
@	Disguise	20	Rifle
£	Good	30	Ammunition
$	Dry	40	Ambush
%	Function	50	War
^	Alive		

Code 11:

G, @, 203 (202 A)

a) A forest can hide many objects
b) The forest hides many women
c) A few women are disguised as trees
d) Lots of men are hiding in the wood
e) Many men are disguised as a forest

Code 12:

30, (202 $), 20, 207, %

a) The rifle does not often work with damp ammunition
b) Damp ammunition seldom works
c) Damp ammunition in the rifle sometimes works
d) A damp rifle often doesn't function
e) Wet ammunition doesn't often work

Code 13:

J, (203 E), (205, £), H

a) Most Spanish soldiers ear good food
b) The Spanish army eats lots of good food
c) Nice food is eaten by many Spanish soldiers
d) Lots of Spanish soldiers eat good food
e) The Spanish army have the best provisions

Code 14:

(203, 10), %, 203 (205, F)

a) Horses do lots of work in the hills
b) Horses are best in the mountains
c) Working horses are in many hills
d) Horses are working in the mountains
e) The hills are where the horses function

Code 15:

@, %, £

a) Camouflage works best
b) Good disguises work well
c) The functioning of the disguise is good
d) The disguise functions particularly well
e) Camouflage works well

Code 16:

203 (L, A, I), 207, (203 F)

a) Many families are on the plain
b) Many families often walk in the hills
c) People are not often in the hills
d) Most families don't walk in the hills
e) People are not usually found in the hills

Code 17:

205 (203 (L, A)), (202, ^), 50

a) Men and women die in war
b) Very many people die in war
c) War kills people
d) Very many people lived through the war
e) The war is so big many people are being killed

Code 18:

E, (202, 204), (208 203), 206 (20, 30)

a) The civilian does not have many weapons
b) The soldier has only one loaded weapon
c) Without many weapons the soldier is nothing
d) The soldier has his loaded weapon
e) Some weapons are not with the soldiers

Code 19:

!, 203 206 (L, 10), B, 40

a) The cavalry prepared many fierce ambushes
b) The men prepared their horses for the fierce ambush
c) The fierce cavalry are ready to ambush
d) Many men and their horses are ready to ambush
e) The men were prepared for the fierce ambush

Code 20:

205 !, (203 E), (205 209), (208 ^), G

a) The fiercest soldiers live in the forest
b) Most often the fierce soldiers live in the forest
c) The forest often contains fierce soldiers
d) Very fierce soldiers commonly die in the forest
e) The most aggressive soldiers usually live in the forest

Code 21:

Which would be the most useful additional code to convey the following?

In war, bombs often cause heavy casualties

a) Contain
b) Explosive
c) Create
d) Death
e) Tragedy

Code 22:

Which would be the most useful additional code to convey the following?

Perhaps the Spanish Cavalry will win the battle

a) Cavalry
b) Battle
c) Maybe
d) Victory
e) Future

Code 23:

Which two codes would be the most useful additional codes to convey the following?

I like to hide my money underneath the mattress

a) Camouflage, Beneath
b) Gold, Mine
c) Coins, Bedding

d) Bed, Conceal
e) Prefer, Money

Code 24:

Choose the best code for the following sentence:

Perhaps the family can be brought together

a) (208, 209) 206, (L, I)
b) 201, 206 (L, A)
c) 206, (L, A, I)
d) (209, 201) (L, A, I), 205
e) 201, (L, A, I), 206

Code 25:

Choose the best code for the following sentence:

The forest is in front of the hills

a) G, 200, (203, F)
b) 200, G, (203, F)
c) G, 205, (203, F)
d) G, 200, F
e) 203, F, 200, G

Code 26:

Choose the best code for the following sentence:

The man has hidden his horses in the wood

a) @, L, 10
b) (203, 10), L, @
c) L, G, 203, 10
d) L, @, G, (203, 10)
e) 10, @, G, 203

Decision Analysis Practice Question Answers:

Code Set 1

Code 1: Answer: e) Gravity keeps the planet in the solar system

Gravity, Contains (Planet, Solar System)
'Contains' can be interpreted as 'keeps in' and is referring to a single planet and the solar system

Code 2: Answer: a) Roll the wheel forward until the slack is taken up by the rope.

Forward Wheel, (Not Stop) (Until Against Rope)
This implies that phrases 'not stop' and 'until against rope' are linked. This phrase is then linked to 'forward wheel' and this is the only explanation that links these

Code 3: Answer: b) Don't expect to be able to breathe on a planet with low gravity.

Expect (Small Air), Planet Is (Small Gravity)
'Small Air' can be interpreted as 'difficult to breathe'.
The coding specifically uses 'expect' and this is not best interpreted as a definitive statement such as in answer a) 'a lack of gravity leads to a lack of air'. Planet is singular, unlike in answers c) and d). Answer e) does not make any sense and does not use the code 'expect'.

Code 4: Answer: a) Expect things to be heavier on a planet with higher gravity.

More Gravity Planet, Expect More Weight
This implies that we should expect more weight on a planet with more gravity and this answer states this well.

Code 5: Answer: a) Bricks are becoming loose under the weight.

Opposite Stop (Loose, Bricks), Underneath Weight
'Opposite Stop' implies 'starting' or 'becoming'. The other answers do not make full or accurate use of all the code.

Code 6: Answer: d) A few animals will become extinct soon

(Opposite Most) Animals, Toward Stop, Forward Time Small
'Opposite most animals' can be interpreted as 'A few animals'. 'Toward stop' can be taken to mean 'are moving toward the end, or extinction' and 'forward time small' translates as 'soon'

Code 7: Answer: d) The largest animals are toughest

Opposite (Most Small), Animals (Most Tough)
The opposite of the 'most small' is the 'most large' or 'largest'
'Most tough' is 'toughest'
The answer c) uses animal in the singular and is not as close an interpretation as the correct answer

Code 8: Answer: e) The animals are becoming thirsty in the wind

(Forward Air), Animals, (Toward Thirsty)
'Forward Air' can be interpreted as 'Wind'
'Toward Thirsty' can be interpreted as 'Becoming thirsty'
The answers a) and c) use all the code but do not make sense

Code 9: Answer: b) The anchor has been washed away

(Lead Weight), Washed (Opposite Toward)
'Opposite Toward' is interpreted as 'Away'
'Lead weight' is interpreted as 'Anchor'
Although this is a somewhat tenuous interpretation, none of the other possible answers are as good.

Code 10: Answer: a) A helium balloon will rise.

True (Helium Balloon Against Gravity)
'Against gravity' can be interpreted as 'rise'. The phrase could be interpreted as 'It is true that a helium balloon will rise' but this is implied in the definitive statement 'A helium balloon will rise'

Code 11: Answer e) The honey is even sweeter this year.

Liquid, (Bees, Opposite Disassemble), (More, Opposite, Sour), Compared (Time back)
'Liquid, (Bees, Opposite Disassemble)' can be interpreted as 'the liquid bees make' or 'honey'
(More, Opposite, Sour) is 'more sweet' or 'sweeter'
'Compared (time back) can be used to turn 'sweeter' to 'even sweeter this year'

Code 12:

Answer: e) Understanding the pathways of pain will help us to reduce suffering.

(Suffer, Less), Method (Disassemble, Pain), (Toward, Explain)
'Toward explain' is interpreted here as 'Understanding', 'Method (Disassemble, Pain)' is 'the pathways of pain'

Code 13: Answer a) I am against the death penalty.

Personal, Generalise, Against (Stop Life) Method (Suspend Rope)
'Suspend rope' can be interpreted as 'hanging'. Answer c) is close but adds in 'most people'. If the answer was simply 'Most people are against hanging' this would be the best answer. Personal should not be used twice as in 'Personal' for 'I' and 'Personal, generalise' for 'Most people'.

Code 14: Answer d) Lead is heavier than helium, probably because it is more affected by gravity.

(More, Weight), (Lead Compared Helium), (Suspect, More, Gravity). This sentence doesn't really make sense in a true physical sense, but this is deliberate. The trick here is to use your reasoning abilities to interpret the codes regardless of your knowledge. In answer c), there is no coding for 'both are equally affected', instead 'more' is coded making this answer unlikely.

Code 15: Answer: b) I think a planet not yet discovered will support life

Personal, Suspect, Unknown, Planet, Life, Allow
There are no hints at linking in this code, so make sure all the code is used as correctly as possible and in as near to the order given as possible:
'Personal, Suspect' can be interpreted as 'I suspect' or 'I think'
'Planet, Unknown' is 'Planet not yet discovered'
'Life, Allow' is 'Will support life'

Code 16: Answer: a) Allow me more of a home life

Personal, Allow, More (Personal Life)
(Personal Life) can be interpreted as 'Home life'
As well as 'I', personal can also be interpreted as 'me'

Code 17: Answer e) Lead can destroy the building blocks of life

Lead, Attack, (Opposite Disassemble), Bricks, Life
(Opposite Disassemble) can be interpreted as 'Assemble' or 'Assembling' or 'Building'. The answer b) is a possible correct answer as 'DNA' could be interpreted as 'A building block of life' but this requires some big jumps in interpretation and the correct answer uses the code with less interpretation required

Code 18: Answer: c) A life full of pain is an unhappy life

Generalise, (Life Contains Pain) (Sour Life)
This is a general statement about 'A life containing pain' and 'an unhappy life' and links the two statements

Code 19: Answer b) Dehydrated animals die quickly

(More Thirsty) Animals, (Opposite Life), (Less Time)
'More Thirsty' can be interpreted as 'Dehydrated' and 'Less Time' as 'Quickly'
All the code is used in order and this answer is correct. In three of the answers the singular of 'Animals' has been used and can be quickly excluded.

Code 20: Answer d) Honey, I can't sleep

(Bees, Liquid), Personal, Attach (Sleep, Less)
(Bees, Liquid) can be interpreted as 'Honey'
Attach (Sleep, Less) can be taken literally to give 'Sleepless'.
'Honey, I, Sleepless' gives 'Honey, I can't sleep'

Code 21: Answer a) Nut

It's very difficult to see anything in the code that could be used to mean 'Nuts'. 'More' and 'Nut' could be used to give 'Nuts'. 'Opposite Loose' could be used to give 'Tight'. 'Wheel' is already in the code, Personal can be used to convey 'I', 'Opposite Blind' could be used for 'Can See'.

Code 22: Answer: d) Advise, Quantity

Advise can be used to code for 'tell'
Quantity can be used to code 'number'
'Without looking' could be 'Stop Allow (Opposite Blind)'
'Correct' can be given by 'True'

Code 23: Answer: b) High, Meadow

'Take' can be coded for by 'Lead'
Animals is in the code
'Up to the' can be 'Toward'
'High' and 'Meadow' combine to be a 'mountain pasture'

Code 24: Answer: d) (O 3), (J 10), P, 5

(Most Weight), (Again Wheel), Not, Tough

Code 25: Answer: b) 4, 6, 14, (H B)

Rope, Loose, Animals, (Toward Above) is the simplest and most succinct coding available to convey the correct meaning.

Code 26: Answer: a) 209, L, N, (208 207)

Personal, Expect, More, (Life Unknown)

Code Set 2

Code 1: Answer: a) The woman loves children

Woman, Love, (Plural, Child)
This uses the correct code in the correct order. The brackets link 'Plural' and 'Child' to make children

Code 2: Answer: d) The Spanish like food

Spanish, (Reduce, Love), Food
(Reduce, Love) can be linked to each other to make 'like', which is less than love.

Code 3: Answer: c) The family is getting bigger

Combine (Man, Woman, Child), Enlarge
Combining 'Man, Woman, Child' gives 'family'

Code 4: Answer: b) I was not ready for the famine

Personal, (Prepared, Opposite), (Food, Without)
The opposite of prepared is unprepared, or 'not ready'. 'Food, Without' can be linked to give famine.

Code 5: Answer: c) We are thirsty

(Plural, Personal), (Without, Liquid)
'Plural' and 'Personal' can be linked to give 'We'. 'Without' and 'Liquid' together gives 'thirsty'.

Code 6: Answer: d) The elderly love the woodland

Plural (Opposite, Child), Love, Forest
The opposite of a child could be an old person.
Many old people are 'the elderly'

Code 7: Answer: b) The fat soldier loved food

(Enlarge, Soldier) (Before, Love), Food
'Enlarge, Soldier' can be taken to mean a 'Large' or 'Fat Soldier'
'Before, Love' can be linked to mean love in the past tense, or 'Loved'

Code 8: Answer: c) Many couples are without water

Combine (Man, Woman), Plural, (Without, Liquid)
Combine (Man, Woman) can be taken to be a 'Couple'. 'Plural' is then used to make 'Many Couples'

Code 9: Answer: e) Our supplies may be heavy

(Enlarge, Personal), Combine (Food, Water), Possibility, Heavy
'Enlarge Personal' is 'Our'. Combine (Food, Water) can be interpreted as 'Supplies'. Possibility gives 'may be'

Code 10: Answer: d) The family is often hungry

Combine (Man, Woman, Child), Common, (Without, Food)
(Combine (Man, Woman, Child) gives 'The family'
(Without, Food) is 'Hungry'

Code 11: Answer: d) Lots of men are hiding in the wood

Forest, Disguise, Plural (Opposite Woman)
This gives a sensible translation using all the code

Code 12: Answer: a) The rifle does not often work with damp ammunition

Ammunition, (Opposite Dry), Rifle, Seldom, Function
This is the only answer that uses all the code and no more, even though the order of the words has been changed.

Code 13: Answer: e) The Spanish army have the best provisions

Spanish, (Plural Soldier), (Enlarge, Good), Food

Code 14: Answer: d) Horses are working in the mountains

(Plural, Horse), Function, Plural (Enlarge, Hill)

Code 15: Answer: e) Camouflage works well

Disguise, Function, Good
'Good' can be used for 'Well'

Code 16: Answer: c) People are not often in the hills

Plural (Man, Woman, Child), Seldom, (Plural Hill)

Code 17: Answer: b) Very many people die in war

Enlarge (Plural (Man, Woman)), (Opposite, Alive), War

Code 18: Answer: b) The soldier has only one loaded weapon

Soldier, (Opposite Without), (Reduce Plural), Combine (Rifle Ammunition)

Code 19: Answer: c) The fierce cavalry are ready to ambush

Fierce, Plural Combine (Man, Horse), Prepared, Ambush

Code 20: Answer: e) The most aggressive soldiers usually live in the forest

Enlarge Fierce, (Plural Soldier), (Enlarge Common), (Reduce Alive), Forest
'Reduce alive' here is used to reduce the length of the word to 'live'

Code 21: Answer: b) Explosive

'War' and 'Heavy' are in the code
'Common' and 'Possibility' could be 'Often' and 'Cause'
'(Opposite Alive) (Plural Soldier)' could be 'casualties

'Bombs' is not easy to code and therefore 'Explosive' is the most useful new code

Code 22: Answer: d) Victory

'Perhaps' can be 'Possibility'
Spanish' is in the code
'Cavalry' can be 'Plural (Combine (Horse, Soldier))'
Battle could be 'Reduce War'
'Victory' could give 'win' which is otherwise hard to code

Code 23: Answer: c) Coins, Bedding

'I' and 'my' can be coded with 'Personal'
'Like' can be 'Reduce love'
'to hide' can be 'disguise'
'Money', 'Underneath' and 'Mattress' are hard to code and two codes for any of these would be useful. 'Coins' and 'Bedding' are used for 'Money' and 'Mattress'

Code 24: Answer: e) 201, (L, A, I), 206

Possibility, (Man, Woman, Child), Combine translates neatly to the required code

Code 25: Answer: a) G, 200, (203, F)

Forest, Before, (Plural, Hill) gives a good succinct code for the message with the code in the most logical order

Code 26: Answer: d) L, @, G, (203, 10)

Man, Disguise, Forest, (Plural, Horse) whilst not in exactly the order of the code has all the necessary words to make the message - none of the others do

Chapter 5

Situational Judgement

Situational Judgement

What is it?

UKCAT says 'The test measures your capacity to understand real world situations and to identify critical factors and appropriate behaviour in dealing with them'

You will be presented with a series of scenarios and then asked to assess the appropriateness or importance of different actions. There will be 20 scenarios each requiring between 3 and 6 responses and a total of 67 items to answer in 27 minutes (including one minute to read the instructions). No medical knowledge is required to answer the scenarios.

You will be asked to rate each action as:

Very appropriate – 'if it addresses at least one aspect of the situation'
Appropriate but not ideal – 'it could be done, but is not necessarily a good thing to do'
Inappropriate but not awful – 'it should not really be done, but would not be terrible'
Very inappropriate – should definitely not be done and would make the situation worse'

Or you will be asked to rate the 'importance' of actions:

Very important – is vital to be taken into account
Important – important but not vital
Of minor importance – could be taken in to account but doesn't really matter
Not important at all – should definitely not be taken in to account

Why is situational judgement included in the test?

Throughout your career you will be required to act with integrity and as part of a team. You will need to be able to stand back and get perspective to be able to take the most appropriate action. You will almost certainly come across these types of questions again - SJTs are widely used for medical selection as part of job applications.

Top tips

Remember you can use each option more than once.
Try and think about what should be done to achieve the best outcome.
Don't think of each option as the only thing that would be done, just whether that action is appropriate or important in relation to the context.

In general, positive actions that will help the situation are 'very appropriate' and anything that may cause harm or make a situation worse is 'very inappropriate'. The greyer areas in between are harder. If something is 'unnecessary but won't cause harm' then it is 'inappropriate but not awful'. If something might be helpful but doesn't completely resolve the problem, then it could be classed as 'appropriate but not ideal'.

Usually, 'explaining' and 'exploring why something has happened' are 'very appropriate things to do.
'Telling' or 'ordering' people to do things is often less appropriate.

Worked Examples

Example 1:

You are in the street just outside your hospital when a woman comes towards you, obviously angry. She wrongly accuses you of having stolen £3 from her bag. Your accommodation is about 100m away.

Decide how appropriate you think the following actions are:

1. Explain politely that she is mistaken and call the police to help her look in to the matter further

2. Tell her that if she does not leave you alone you will call the police

3. Run as fast as you can home and ask your friends to help barricade the door

4. Explain that you were not responsible, that you were elsewhere when the money was stolen and offer any assistance you can.

Answers:

Explain politely that she is mistaken and call the police to help her look in to the matter further

Appropriate but not ideal. If money has been stolen, then the police could be involved. However, this is a trivial amount and it is worth exploring other possibilities first. Perhaps she has lost the money or it has fallen from her bag? It is important you explain politely that you were not to blame.

Tell her that if she does not leave you alone you will call the police

Very inappropriate This should be a situation that you are able to defuse yourself, without involvement of the police. She is obviously angry, but there is no evidence that you are feeling threatened and if you threaten to call the police, you will only antagonize the situation.

Run as fast as you can home and ask your friends to barricade the door

Very inappropriate Again, this is not how a responsible adult would behave and makes you appear childish and possibly guilty of the crime. This course of action does nothing to improve the situation.

Explain politely that you were not responsible, that you were elsewhere when she says the money was stolen and offer any assistance you can.

Very appropriate This proves you were not responsible and you are attempting to ease the situation by offering to help.

Example 2:

As a medical student, you take part in a consultant-led ward round, visiting 15 patients on the orthopaedic ward. You will be asked to examine some of the patients. How important do you rate the following?

1. Dressing smartly

2. Washing hands between each patient

3. Taking a 10-minute break after two hours to have a drink

208

4. Making sure that all questions you have about patient care are answered during the ward round

Answers

Dressing smartly

Important However, patient care is not going to suffer if your shirt is hanging out.

Washing hands between each patient

Very important This is vital as you are likely to spread bacteria if you do not do this. It is very important to remain clean during the round, particularly after examining patients.

Taking a 10-minute break after two hours to have a drink

Of minor importance After two hours you may be tired and a break may help you learn better

Making sure that all questions you have about patient care are answered during the ward round

Of minor importance You will almost certainly have many questions. However, the ward round may not be the place to ask all of them.

Situational Judgement Exercise

Scenario 1:

As part of second year at medical school, students are offered a placement for 'special study'. Richard is assigned to anaesthetics but makes it obvious he would much rather be doing general surgery as he wishes to be a surgeon. Unfortunately the surgical special study group is full. The other members of his group are starting to find his attitude and behaviour disruptive.

How appropriate are the following actions by the anaesthetics tutor?

1. Reassigning Richard to a surgical group, despite it being full

2. Addressing the group as a whole and asking them to try and work more effectively together

3. Discussing with Richard alone that he needs to improve his behaviour

4. Do nothing

5. Refer the matter to the dean of the medical school

Scenario 2:

Whilst working as a student on a GP placement, you take blood from a 22-year-old man. During the procedure he begins to feel faint and looks clammy.

How appropriate are the following actions you could take?

6. Continue the procedure and try to finish it quickly

7. Stop the procedure immediately and call for help

8. Stop the procedure and ask him to come back another time to complete it

9. Stop the procedure and discuss the event with the GP

10. Stop the procedure, ask the patient to lie down and try again.

Scenario 3:

Nusa is a fourth year medical student. Whilst waiting at a bus stop, and late for an important exam, an elderly man next to her in the queue clutches his chest, collapses to the floor and loses consciousness. The bus arrives just after Nusa has called the ambulance and has started giving chest compressions.

How appropriate are the following actions?

11. Explain the situation to one of the passengers and ask them to take over compressions so she can get on the bus

12. Ignore the bus and continue compressions until the ambulance arrives

13. Ask the bus driver to wait and if possible provide help with the resuscitation

14. Stop compressions as very few people survive out-of-hospital cardiac arrests

Scenario 4:

Julia is a nurse on the medical admissions ward. It is alleged by one of the other nurses that she has signed an X-ray - request form with the signature of one of the doctors.

How appropriate do you consider the following actions by the hospital?

15. Relieving Julia of her post with immediate effect

16. Reporting Julia to the nursing and midwifery council

17. Interviewing other members of staff working in the ward

18. Reviewing all the patients that Julia has been involved with in the last year

19. Checking with the doctor that she has signed all the forms that have come through in her name

Scenario 5:

Benoit is a French medical student on an exchange in the UK. He has been paired with you and a senior doctor asks him to take a history from a patient whilst he sees another patient. It quickly becomes clear that Benoit's English is not good enough and that he does not fully understand what the patient is saying. Benoit is embarrassed and clearly struggling.

How appropriate are the following actions you could take?

20. Do nothing – the senior doctor has asked Benoit to do this and he should be left to do it to his best ability

21. Take over from Benoit and write the history down for him so he can read it to the senior doctor

22. Help Benoit with the parts of the history that he does not understand and explain the situation to the senior doctor when he returns

23. Call the hospital translation service and ask them to come and help

24. Explain the situation to the clinical tutor and ask a fluent French-speaking fellow student to take your place

Answers:

Scenario 1

1. Very inappropriate. If the surgical group is full, adding an extra person may well be detrimental for people already in the surgical group.
2. Very appropriate. Addressing everyone in the group gives them all responsibility to help find a way of working together.
3. Very appropriate. Richard needs to address his behaviour and attitude and talking to him alone will give him the chance to air his views and explain why his wishes cannot be accommodated this time.
4. Very inappropriate. Ignoring the situation will likely lead to it getting worse for the whole group.
5. Appropriate but not ideal. It would be better if an attempt were made to deal with the situation without escalating it to the level of the dean. However, there may have been previous problems and it may be helpful for the dean to be aware of the situation.

Scenario 2

6. Very inappropriate. This is likely to make the situation worse and possibly cause harm to the patient.
7. Very appropriate. This is the best immediate action to take.
8. Very appropriate. The procedure needs to be done so you should ask him to come back.
9. Very appropriate. The GP needs to be aware of the situation
10. Inappropriate but not awful. As a student, if you run in to difficulties you should stop what you are doing and seek help. The action here is unlikely to cause the patient significant harm but is inappropriate.

Scenario 3

11. Very inappropriate. This is a life and death situation. As a fourth year student you will be familiar with resuscitation techniques and should continue until the ambulance arrives, despite your important exam!
12. Very appropriate. Your priority is the collapsed man.
13. Very appropriate. This may also solve your problem of getting to your exam. Although the bus driver may not be skilled in resuscitation, he may be able to help under your supervision and may even have a first aid qualification.
14. Very inappropriate. You are this man's best chance of survival and you should not be making the decision to stop compressions whilst a student.

Scenario 4

15. Very inappropriate. This is an allegation and it would be unfair to sack Julia without investigation. It may however be prudent to remove her from clinical duties for a short while for an investigation as there are concerns regarding patient safety here (potentially inappropriate exposure to X-rays).
16. Very inappropriate. This is an allegation and at present this would be inappropriate.
17. Very appropriate. Some form of investigation needs to take place.
18. Very inappropriate. At this stage, with this level of concern, this would be an over reaction and waste people's time.
19. Very appropriate. This would form part of an investigation in to this allegation.

20. Very inappropriate. This would be unproductive and humiliating for Benoit.
21. Inappropriate but not awful. This would save Benoit's embarrassment but would not help him in the future.
22. Very appropriate. Explaining the situation to the doctor may help solve the problem for Benoit in the future.
23. Very inappropriate. This would be an inappropriate use of the translation service and there are better ways of resolving the situation.
24. Very appropriate. This would make Benoit's trip much more useful for him.

Situational Judgement Practice Questions

1. You are a third year medical student. One night your friend comes to you at 3AM in tears. You are aware she has been struggling with her studies and has missed a couple of deadlines recently. She tells you that she has been diagnosed with depression and is now taking medication that appears to be helping. She has an important essay due in tomorrow but says that she is not going to be able to finish it.

Decide whether the following actions are 'very appropriate', 'appropriate but not ideal', 'inappropriate but not awful' or 'very inappropriate':

1. Tell her that she can borrow your essay to help her complete hers on time.

2. Ring the medical tutor at home and ask him to come and talk to her.

3. Advise her to go to sleep and deal with the problem in the morning.

4. Explain that although you feel sorry for her, there is really nothing you can do to help. She will have to deal with the consequences of her chaotic life.

5. Advise her to ring the tutor in the morning and explain the situation.

6. Advise her to go and see her GP and ask for a note for extenuating circumstances.

2. As a final year medical student you travel to Malawi for a medical elective in obstetrics and gynaecology. On arrival at the hospital, you find that you are on the rota as a junior doctor and will be doing three weeks of nights on the delivery suite and three weeks in the neonatal department. The hospital director says that you will be expected to work unsupervised as a doctor as they are currently understaffed.

Decide whether the following actions are 'very appropriate', 'appropriate but not ideal', 'inappropriate but not awful' or 'very inappropriate':

1. Advise the director that you are unqualified for this position and will be looking for an elective experience elsewhere.

2. Discuss with the director the level of supervision that you will have.

3. Thank the director for his confidence in you and accept the post.

4. Discuss the situation with your supervisor in the UK.

5. Agree to take on the position but reassess after a week.

6. Offer to help in the hospital where you can but advise the director that your experience is limited and nights are unacceptable.

3. As a first year medical student you join the university rugby club. You are asked attend a special party for new team recruits where you will have to complete a 'challenge'. Last year you know that several students got into trouble after they were asked to drink 8 pints of beer, run naked down the street and steal a university painting.

Decide whether the following actions are 'very appropriate', 'appropriate but not ideal', 'inappropriate but not awful' or 'very inappropriate':

1. Complete whatever challenge is set to become accepted as a 'good sport' and part of the team.

2. Asking the captain to consider changing the challenge so that you do not have to break the law.

3. Decline the invitation and choose another sport.

4. Tell the captain that you are not feeling well and can't make the party.

4. The medical director of the university hospital is asked to take part in an interview for the local television news agency. There has been an outbreak of gastroenteritis and half the hospital wards have been shut; operating has been suspended.

Decide whether the following are 'very important', 'important', of minor importance' or 'not important at all':

1. The invitation for an interview is accepted by the hospital.

2. The medical director himself gives the interview rather than delegating to his deputy.

3. The medical director apologises for the outbreak to the public.

4. The news team is allowed to film inside the shut hospital wards so the public can see the extent of the problem.

5. The medical director gives a definitive timescale for reopening the wards.

5. As a first year medical student you attend operating theatres and watch the removal of a colorectal cancer from a 50-year old woman. Afterwards you go to see her on the ward and realise that she is a friend of your mother's. You think that she probably didn't recognise you as she was still a little sleepy from the anaesthetic.

Decide whether the following actions are 'very appropriate', 'appropriate but not ideal', 'inappropriate but not awful' or 'very inappropriate':

1. Telephone your mother and ask her to go and see her friend in hospital, explaining that she has not been well but giving no details.

2. Go back later to see the patient and see how she has fared, explaining that you are the daughter of a family friend.

3. Say nothing to anyone regarding your personal connection to the patient and try not to see her again.

4. Send the patient a 'get-well' card and visit them in a few days.

6. Whilst working as an F1 doctor on your surgical rotation, you see a man arguing with one of your patients. He then reaches into the patient's drawer and removes her purse and walks off the ward carrying it.

Decide whether the following actions are 'very appropriate', 'appropriate but not ideal', 'inappropriate but not awful' or 'very inappropriate':

1. Dial 999 and then hospital security and ask them to detain the man.

2. Ask the patient what has just happened and if they need any assistance.

3. Do nothing – this was a private conversation and there is plenty of work to do.

4. Discuss the situation with the ward clerk, who also saw the event, and then decide whether to call the police or not.

5. Contact your consultant and ask her what she thinks you should do.

7. You are a third year medical student. In the middle of winter, you are walking home from the hospital alone in the dark. You are mugged and your bag is taken. Unfortunately you were carrying a notebook that had some confidential information regarding patients in it and this has been taken.

Decide whether the following actions are 'very appropriate', 'appropriate but not ideal', 'inappropriate but not awful' or 'very inappropriate':

1. Call the police, explain the situation and ask them to prioritise the case.

2. Say nothing to anyone at the hospital for 24 hours until the police have had a chance to track the bag down.

3. Try and make a list of all the patients who might be affected and go back to the hospital the next day and speak to them individually, explaining what has happened and how sorry you are.

4. Advise the hospital management team what has happened and ask for their help in dealing with the situation.

8. On the first day of his medical rotation as a student at the hospital, Jim wakes up, feels sick, vomits and has two episodes of diarrhoea. The dean of

the medical school has emphasised how important it is that everyone makes the first day as there will be a lot of teaching that will not be repeated.

Decide whether the following actions are 'very appropriate', 'appropriate but not ideal', 'inappropriate but not awful' or 'very inappropriate':

1. Visit the pharmacy, take some anti-sickness medication and attend the first day of his rotation.

2. Ask one of his friends to sign him in and make sure he catches up another day.

3. Phone the medical student office and explain what has happened.

4. Rest at home for the rest of the day.

5. Ask a friend to explain to the dean that he is unwell and unfortunately cannot attend.

9. During the end-of-year exams in her second year at medical school, Rachel receives news that her father has died suddenly from a heart attack.

Decide whether the following are 'very important', 'important', of minor importance' or 'not important at all':

1. Staying on and completing the exams so as not to fail the year

2. Discussing the situation with the dean of the medical school

3. Returning home to see her mother as soon as possible

4. Attending the funeral, even though it clashes with an important end-of-year exam

5. Trying to put the situation out of her mind whilst she completes her exams

10. While walking along the street Rachel sees an old man lying on the pavement. His walking frame is lying to one side. She approaches and asks what the problem is. He tells her he has 'no problem' and asks her to 'go away'. She notices that he has a bruise on the side of his head and a bleeding nose.

Decide whether the following actions are 'very appropriate', 'appropriate but not ideal', 'inappropriate but not awful' or 'very inappropriate':

1. She respects what the man has asks her to do and leaves him alone

2. She makes sure that he is comfortable and then leaves him

3. She calls 999 and arranges for an ambulance to come immediately

4. She calls the non-emergency number for the police and asks them to deal with the situation

5. She keeps a safe distance and tries to obtain more details about what has happened to him

11. In the hospital canteen Greg, a third year medical student, overhears two doctors sitting on the next table discussing a patient. They are discussing the difficulties they had controlling Mr Anderson the night before when he 'went nuts' and hit one of the nurses because he thought she was a 'Nazi' and that he was back in a concentration camp.

Decide whether the following actions are 'very appropriate', 'appropriate but not ideal', 'inappropriate but not awful' or 'very inappropriate':

1. Greg advises the two doctors that he can hear them discussing a patient and that they are breaching patient confidentiality

2. Greg asks the doctors to talk about something else as he is trying to eat his lunch and not think about work for a bit

3. Greg asks them how they managed to control the situation in the end and learns something from them for future use

4. Greg advises the two doctors that he will be reporting them to the hospital authorities as they have breached patient confidentiality

5. Greg takes the doctors names and contacts the General Medical Council for advice on how to deal with the situation

12. Hassan, a 24-year-old Syrian medical student is on an exchange at the local hospital. Whilst talking to a 50 year old man who has had a heart attack, the man says to him 'I don't want no foreign doctor treating me in Britain.'

Decide whether the following actions are 'very appropriate', 'appropriate but not ideal', 'inappropriate but not awful' or 'very inappropriate':

1. Hassan ignores the comment and carries on taking a history

2. Hassan explains where he is from and the training that he has had

3. Hassan walks away from the situation without saying anything and asks another doctor to see the patient

4. Hassan attempts to discuss with the man the reasons for his prejudices

5. Hassan advises the man that he is in no situation to be picky and that if he makes further racist comments security will be called and he will be removed from the hospital

13. On a hospital night out as an F2 doctor, you see one of your consultants drink a couple of bottles of wine. Half an hour later, he gets in his car and begins his drive home.

Decide whether the following actions are 'very appropriate', 'appropriate but not ideal', 'inappropriate but not awful' or 'very inappropriate':

1. Deciding not to call the police - the future career of the consultant and care of his patients will be jeopardised.

2. Calling the police if the consultant drives his car home

3. Attempting to stop the consultant from driving home if it is safe to do so

4. Discussing the situation with the chief executive of the hospital the next day

5. Confront the consultant regarding the inappropriateness of his actions at work the next day

14. During the final exams of medical school, you hear a rumour that the pathology paper is available on line and has the answers with it.

Decide whether the following actions are 'very appropriate', 'appropriate but not ideal', 'inappropriate but not awful' or 'very inappropriate':

1. Ignore the rumour and sit the paper as planned

2. Email the chief examiner regarding the rumour you have heard

3. Check out the site so that no-one else has an unfair advantage

4. Inform the exam invigilator when you arrive to take the exam

15. You are a first year medical student. Your mother's friend has just been diagnosed with SLE and has asked if she can chat with you about her condition. You have not yet covered it at medical school.

Decide whether the following actions are 'very appropriate', 'appropriate but not ideal', 'inappropriate but not awful' or 'very inappropriate':

1. Advising your mother that you have not yet covered the subject at medical school and decline to talk to her.

2. Advise your mother that it is inappropriate and to tell her friend that you are busy.
3. Read as much as you can about the subject and then offer to help the friend with her research about the disease.

4. Ask your mother to remind her friend that you are still a medical student and ask her to see her GP for further information.

16. The head consultant in a busy accident and emergency is trying to improve the working environment in her department. Staff are stretched and morale is low. The busiest period of the year – Christmas – is four weeks away.

Decide whether the following actions are 'very appropriate', 'appropriate but not ideal', 'inappropriate but not awful' or 'very inappropriate':

1. Set each member of staff targets to reach with penalties if they do not reach them.

2. Meet with the head of the nursing department and ask for her opinion on how to improve conditions.

3. Advise members of staff that they will be watched closely over the next few weeks. Any members of staff not pulling their weight will be dealt with.

4. Contact the media and ask them to tell people to see their GP rather than coming to A and E inappropriately.

5. Liaise with the human resources department and ask for extra cover during the busy period.

6. Threaten to resign unless managers start funding the department properly.

7. Call a departmental meeting, explain to everyone that the busiest time of the year is coming and ask for ideas to help ease the situation.

17. You are a first year doctor and your colleague is away on sick leave, leaving you to cover the ward and do the jobs alone. At half past four, it becomes obvious to you that there are several hours worth of work to do.

Decide whether the following actions are 'very appropriate', 'appropriate but not ideal', 'inappropriate but not awful' or 'very inappropriate':

1. You stay until all the work is completed, otherwise there will be more to do tomorrow and patient care may suffer.

2. You leave at five o'clock as planned – you are due to meet a friend that evening and would otherwise be late.

3. You contact the consultant and explain you have to leave at five o'clock.

4. Prioritize which jobs need to be done that day and which can wait.

5. Enlist the help of a fellow junior doctor and return the favour another day.

6. Phone up your colleague, find out how sick they are and ask them to come in and help for a couple of hours.

18. It is Saturday and you are working in the hospital as a junior doctor covering the wards. Unexpectedly, the computer system suddenly goes down – there is no access to blood results, patient lists or x-rays. Without all of these it is

difficult to do your job. The IT department ring and say that they are working as fast as they can but it will be an hour before the computers are working again.

Decide whether the following actions are 'very appropriate', 'appropriate but not ideal', 'inappropriate but not awful' or 'very inappropriate':

1. Take the opportunity to have a break and go for a coffee.

2. Ask the nursing staff whether there are any jobs that you could be getting on with.

3. Quickly check that the patients are in no danger and make a note of any problems with a pencil and paper.

4. Telephone the IT department and ask them to hurry as you have important clinical work to get on with and patients may suffer if you are held up.

5. Fill out an 'incident form' and make a formal complaint to the managers regarding the inadequacy of the computing system.

19. A hospital manager has been involved with interviewing for a new chief executive to the local hospital trust - the person in overall charge of the running of the hospital. Four people applied, including two from the present management team of the hospital. One of the internal applicants has been appointed to the job and the other, Richard Thomas, comes to the hospital manager complaining that 'they should have got the job and that the process has been unfair'.

Decide whether the following actions are 'very appropriate', 'appropriate but not ideal', 'inappropriate but not awful' or 'very inappropriate':

1. The manager listens to what Richard has to say.

2. The manager advises Richard that the decision is final and due process has been followed.

3. The manager advises the successful applicant that Richard is very upset not to have the job.

4. The manager offers Richard a cup of tea, lets him have a grumble and says how sorry he is he didn't get the job.

5. The manager advises Richard of the reasons why he did not get the job – that he was felt to have relatively poor inter-personal skills and be less of a team player.

20. Whilst a third year medical student, three applicants from your old college have contacted you to ask for help preparing for their interviews. You give them some brief general advice on good interview technique. Shortly afterwards, the medical school asks you to help with interviews for prospective medical students.

Decide whether the following actions are 'very appropriate', 'appropriate but not ideal', 'inappropriate but not awful' or 'very inappropriate':

1. You advise the medical school that you know three of the applicants and have had contact with them to help them prepare for their interviews.

2. You advise the medical school that you are unable to help.

3. You say nothing and help with the interviews, but make sure you are fair with the applicants that you know.

4. Email the applicants you know so that they are aware that you may be interviewing them.

Situational Judgement Practice Question Answers

Reminder: The answers here are, by nature, debatable and are the considered opinion of the authors. No doubt you will disagree with some!

Very appropriate – 'if it addresses at least one aspect of the situation'
Appropriate but not ideal – 'it could be done, but is not necessarily a good thing to do'
Inappropriate but not awful – 'it should not really be done, but would not be terrible'
Very inappropriate – should definitely not be done and would make the situation worse'

Very important – is vital to be taken into account
Important – important but not vital
Of minor importance – could be taken in to account but doesn't really matter
Not important at all – should definitely not be taken in to account.

1.
    1. **Very inappropriate.** Encouraging her to plagiarise your work will make the situation worse.
    2. **Very inappropriate.** At 3AM, there is no need to do this – if necessary she should ring the tutor in the morning.
    3. **Very appropriate.** At 3AM, her priority is sleep and she is unlikely to complete the essay now.
    4. **Very inappropriate.** This is likely to upset her more.
    5. **Very appropriate.** This will allow resolution of the problem one way or another.
    6. **Appropriate but not ideal.** This might be appropriate if her mental health issues have contributed to her not being able to complete her essay. However, we have no evidence of this in the information given – 'the medication is helping'.

2.
    1. **Appropriate but not ideal.** There has clearly been a miscommunication here. You have been given duties that you are not ready for and could be a danger to patients. However, there may be other ways to resolve the problem such as asking for different duties and helping within your capabilities.
    2. **Very appropriate.** This may resolve the problem and you may find a role that suits your capabilities.
    3. **Very inappropriate.** You should not accept a post that will not provide the support you need and may lead to patient harm.
    4. **Very appropriate.** They may be able to help and may have come across this situation before.
    5. **Very inappropriate.** The director is clear in what is expected – and you are not ready for this post.
    6. **Inappropriate but not awful.** You should expect to help as required – at night if that is their wish, but you should have an appropriate level of supervision.

3.
    1. **Very inappropriate.** You could jeopardise your career if the challenge is anything like last years!
    2. **Inappropriate but not awful.** You may still be pressured in to something you do not want to do.

3. **Inappropriate but not awful.** You should not have to change your sport simply because of this problem.
4. **Inappropriate but not awful.** Lying to protect yourself and your career is not the right thing to do, but is not 'awful'.

4.
1. **Very important.** The shutting of half the hospital wards is of vital importance to the local community. Communication with the community by a member of the hospital team and explaining the situation is very important.
2. **Important.** This is not vital, but would be appropriate given the level of seriousness of the situation.
3. **Of minor importance.** This may go some way to defusing the likely anger in the local community. However, the director should not apologise for a situation that the hospital may not have had any control over.
4. **Not important at all.** This may be counter-productive and lead to spreading of the disease.
5. **Not important at all.** This should not be done as it cannot be done accurately. Raising expectations, only for them not to be met, would make the situation worse.

5.
1. **Very inappropriate.** This would be breaking patient confidentiality. You should not even reveal that your mother's friend has been in hospital – she may not want anyone to know.
2. **Very appropriate.** This shows compassion and allows you to reassure the patient that you will not break her confidentiality.
3. **Inappropriate but not awful.** This will not cause harm to the patient, but will also not cause any benefit to the patient. There is no reason to take this course of action.
4. **Appropriate but not ideal.** This might lead the patient to worry about confidentiality, for example, how did you know they were there? It would be better to take them a get-well card personally.

6.
1. **Very inappropriate.** Without further information, this may make the situation worse – you have no evidence that the man is stealing the purse and he may be going to the shop to buy something for the patient.
2. **Very appropriate.**
3. **Very inappropriate.** If you witness possible harm to your patient, you should do something about it.
4. **Very inappropriate.** Without asking the patient, you will both be speculating as to what has happened.

5. **Inappropriate but not awful.** You should be able to work this one out yourself without bothering your consultant!

7.
1. **Appropriate but not ideal.** You need to contact the police and explain the situation. However, they will decide how to prioritise the case.
2. **Very inappropriate.** You need to tell the hospital as soon as possible so that the appropriate personnel can decide what action may be necessary.
3. **Very inappropriate.** Trying to handle this situation yourself will only land you in further trouble and cause more worry to the patients involved.
4. **Very appropriate.** This is the best course of action.

8.
1. **Very inappropriate.** Jim is potentially infectious. No matter how important the teaching, introducing a diarrhoea and vomiting bug to the hospital is inacceptable.
2. **Very inappropriate.** Jim should not lie. He has a good reason not to be in attendance.
3. **Very appropriate.**
4. **Very appropriate.**
5. **Appropriate but not ideal**. Jim should do this himself.

9.
1. **Not important at all.** This is a time to mourn and be at home with the rest of the family. Some things are more important than exams, and universities should generally be able to cope with genuine emergencies such as this. Rachel is unlikely to have to re-do the year.
2. **Very important.**
3. **Very important.**
4. **Very important**
5. **Not important at all.** This will be very difficult, is likely to affect her grades and not appropriate action to take.

10.
1. **Very inappropriate.** In most situations it is very appropriate to respect what people ask. However, in this situation it is difficult to tell what the problem is with this man who appears to be extremely vulnerable and in need of assistance. It warrants a little more investigation and the consequences of walking away from an elderly man with a head injury could be dire.
2. **Appropriate but not ideal**. Ensuring that the man is comfortable is good and implies that Rachel makes an assessment of the severity of

his injuries, but it would be better to wait until help arrives, rather than leaving him alone. This could be nearby if he is insistent that Rachel leaves or she feels in danger.

3. **Inappropriate but not awful.** This may be useful, but we cannot tell without further assessment.
4. **Inappropriate but not awful.** The police will be able to organise appropriate help but this could be done by Rachel.
5. **Very appropriate.** This is a situation where more details are needed to make the right decision. Obtaining more details at a safe distance ensures everyone is safe.

11.

1. **Very appropriate.** This will resolve the immediate situation of on-going breach of patient confidentiality.
2. **Inappropriate but not awful.** This makes Greg sound a bit odd but may reduce any further confidentiality issue.
3. **Very inappropriate.** This causes on-going breach of confidentiality.
4. **Inappropriate but not awful.** This is causing an escalation of a fairly minor situation. If the two doctors were to continue following a 'quick word' then this would be more appropriate.
5. **Very inappropriate.** This is heavy handed when simply a quick word will remind the doctors of their confidentiality breach and cause them to cease.

12.

1. **Inappropriate but not awful.** This may be the easiest way for Hassan to cope with the racial slur and continue to learn as a student. However, it does nothing to address the underlying issue of racism, which Hassan should not have to tolerate.
2. **Very appropriate.** This is an attempt by Hassan to address the man's prejudices and may improve the situation.
3. **Appropriate but not ideal.** Hassan can ask someone else to see the patient but nothing is done to challenge the patient's racism.
4. **Very appropriate.** Challenging the man's prejudices may change the way he thinks in the future.
5. **Very inappropriate.** This is an empty threat and although Hassan may feel this way, threatening patients is never appropriate.

13.

1. **Very inappropriate.** Events are moving quickly. The consultant could end is career if he is caught drink-driving. However, far more important is the fact that he could kill himself or someone else on the roads. The career prospects of the consultant should not affect your decision to call the police if you cannot stop him.

2. **Very appropriate.** This must be done as he is a danger to other road users.
3. **Very appropriate.** This would prevent injury to others and also save the consultant's career.
4. **Appropriate but not ideal.** This would lead to action being taken. Ideally someone more senior would help with this.
5. **Inappropriate but not awful.** Confronting the consultant yourself is unlikely to resolve the issue – it would be most appropriate to involve a senior colleague and let them take further action.

14.
1. **Appropriate but not ideal.** This is only a rumour – you do not know for sure. However, you may be at an unfair disadvantage and others may be cheating, so it would be more appropriate to take some action.
2. **Very appropriate.** This allows action to be taken.
3. **Very inappropriate.** This is cheating.
4. **Inappropriate but not awful.** This is too late for anything to be done, but at least the authorities know what has happened and action may be taken at a later date.

15.
1. **Inappropriate but not awful.** This is the truth, but you are probably able to offer some help as to where to find further information. You could also do some research first and share what you have learnt.
2. **Very inappropriate.** There is no need to lie about your lack of knowledge.
3. **Very appropriate.** A good learning opportunity for you.
4. **Appropriate but not ideal.** This ducks the issue and lands the work with someone else.

16.
1. **Inappropriate but not awful.** Setting targets might help some people, but penalties will make low moral even lower.
2. **Very appropriate.** This will make the head nurse feel valued and may come up with some solutions.
3. **Very inappropriate.** Intimidating staff is likely to reduce morale further and be counterproductive. The staff are not the reason the department is busy – it is coming up to Christmas.
4. **Inappropriate but not awful.** This is seeking to blame patients for the department being busy. However, there may be some truth in it and diverting patients to GPs, if done appropriately, would be beneficial to both patients and the department.
5. **Very appropriate.**

6. **Inappropriate but not awful.** This may lead to action, but it may leave the consultant looking silly if no extra resources are found and he does not resign. It's probably better to use this as a last resort!
7. **Very appropriate.** This brings everyone on board and involves and empowers them in the decision-making.

17.

1. **Inappropriate but not awful.** This ensures the patient safety but leaves the junior doctor tired and annoyed. If there is another solution it should be used.
2. **Very inappropriate.** Unfortunately, the friend is going to have to wait. As a professional, your first duty is your patients and you need to find a way to look after them.
3. **Very inappropriate.** For a more important reason it may be appropriate to let a senior know that you have to leave. However, you should be looking for another way to manage the problem and not bother your consultant with this matter.
4. **Very appropriate.** This is crucial.
5. **Very appropriate.** Asking for help when you need it and helping others when they need it is an important part of your future professional career.
6. **Very inappropriate.** You should trust your colleague to make that judgement and not ask them to come in when they are sick.

18.

1. **Very appropriate.** If you are unable to do your work effectively, it is worth using the opportunity to rest. Leaving the hospital for an hour would be unacceptable, but having a short opportunistic break is appropriate.
2. **Very appropriate.** This may be a good way of using your time.
3. **Very appropriate.** This ensures that your patients are safe.
4. **Inappropriate but not awful.** This would be annoying to the IT department and would not cause any benefit, but it would not cause harm.
5. **Very inappropriate.** Venting steam like this is unnecessary and the managers will already be aware of the situation. If it were to keep happening, then this may be appropriate, but the key word here is 'unexpectedly'.

19.

1. **Very appropriate.** Richard is part of the team and can be expected to feel hurt. Letting him vent his feelings is a good way of helping him come to terms with not getting the job.
2. **Very appropriate.** Richard needs to know that it is pointless complaining to enable him to stop brooding and get on with his job.

3. **Inappropriate but not awful.** The successful applicant will probably already be aware of this. However, it may help them to know to tread carefully around Richard for a while. On the other hand, this could be considered as undermining Richard and he may be upset if this were to happen.
4. **Very inappropriate.** This undermines the person who has been successful, although it may be an easy way out for the manager.
5. **Appropriate but not ideal.** This may be true but it is not what Richard needs to hear right now and will upset him even more. He needs the feedback but it would be worth waiting until he has calmed down.

20.
1. **Very appropriate.** The medical school can then decide how you should be involved in the interviews. There is nothing wrong in helping people prepare but to interview them as well would clearly be a conflict of interest.
2. **Very inappropriate.** Without giving reasons this appears odd and unhelpful.
3. **Very inappropriate.** There is a clear conflict of interest and the candidate's places may be jeopardised if you are found out.
4. **Very inappropriate.** You should not let the possibility of interviewing them happen at all.